Responsible National Health Insurance

Mark V. Pauly, Patricia Danzon,
Paul J. Feldstein, and John Hoff

The AEI Press

Publisher for the American Enterprise Institute
WASHINGTON, D.C.

1992

Distributed by arrangement with

University Press of America, Inc.
4720 Boston Way   3 Henrietta Street
Lanham, Md. 20706   London WC2E 8LU England

1 3 5 7 9 10 8 6 4 2

ISBN 0-8447-7016-7 (alk. paper)
ISBN 0-8447-7014-0 (pbk: alk. paper)

Printed in the United States of America

Contents

1
Introduction

National health insurance is again the subject of vigorous debate. The issue is driven by a broad variety of cross-cutting and sometimes inconsistent aspirations: increasingly strident demands to control costs; rhetorical, if not political, demands to cover the uninsured; recognition of the need to cure the inefficiencies of the health care delivery system; and fears of the insured that they may lose their insurance if they change jobs or become sick.

Any plan for reform should be grounded on the fundamental principles on which Americans generally agree. We believe there is agreement that the health care system and the financing of it should be structured in a way that promotes efficiency and equity.

Most of the proposed solutions explicitly espouse a dominant role for government in providing health insurance and in regulating any private insurance that remains. These proposals, like versions of national health insurance that have been proposed for decades, assume that increased and substantial government involvement in the health care system is necessary to guarantee insurance coverage for all Americans and to determine the appropriate allocation of resources to health care expenditures. Our view, in contrast, is that many forms of increased government intervention will make matters worse and that government can ensure equity and promote efficiency not by increasing its role in financing and regulation but by rethinking the nature of government intervention and targeting it to what is necessary to achieve efficiency and equity. Our plan combines governmental assurance of universal coverage with financial assistance as needed to achieve this coverage, in an institutional framework that encourages a vigorously competitive market. We believe this scheme would best achieve the objectives of efficiency and equity. A market enables all persons to act on their quite different desires for health care and forms of

1

health insurance, and their willingness to forgo other goods and services for health care, should they choose to do so. This approach promotes efficiency in the production of health care and health insurance and the proper allocation of resources to health care. Financial assistance tied to the cost to families of obtaining coverage, in place of an open-ended tax exclusion, promotes equity and efficiency.

We assume that it is desirable to preserve, insofar as possible, private markets in health insurance and health care when they work reasonably well and, where they do not, to develop structures that will permit them to do so. People can differ about what is meant by "reasonably well." Where government is less imperfect than markets, we think government should act, but our approach is to prefer markets first and to turn to government only as needed to make markets work well. In this sense our approach is "market oriented"; we would like to design systems, even for health services, in which markets can work, but we are not naively attached to the ideal competitive market in total disregard of reality. We simply take markets as the place to begin. Our objective then is to outline the best possible plan that uses a market-based approach. We have addressed this objective without making assumptions about political feasibility (or someone's conjecture about it), since we think that discussion is best served by first specifying what must be done to apply the principles that we think Americans share and then judging how to implement those principles in an acceptable way.

In this book we first present the outline of the Responsible National Health Insurance (RNHI) concept, following the approach that we took in an article in the spring 1991 issue of *Health Affairs*.[1] Then we turn to matters of implementation and distribution. The actual amounts of coverage, the credits that people of different incomes should receive, and the form of tax financing are choices we leave to the political process. We provide preliminary cost estimates of some sample RNHI plans. For many versions of the plan that we think would be acceptable, the gross cost is in a range that can be easily covered by recycling the amount now spent on Medicaid and the exclusion of employer-paid premiums from federal taxation. These versions of the RNHI can be financed with no increase in federal or state tax rates. We do not mean to imply that our examples necessarily correspond to the voters' desires, but they will serve to outline some options. The political process, reflecting society's judgment, can select from these and other options, based on the political decision of how the relative benefits and burdens should be distributed.

2

First Principles— Efficiency and Equity

Efficiency has two important dimensions: (1) minimizing the cost of whatever services are provided; and (2) choosing the level, quality, and mixture of health services, relative to other goods and services, that lead to the greatest excess of benefits over costs. Incorporating the need to balance quality and cost, efficiency reflects choices in which the resources used to furnish goods and services yield maximum value to consumers.

An efficient system does not necessarily have the lowest cost. The most cost-constraining system is the one that incurs no cost. This obviously is not desirable. Nor is a strategy that has contained costs in other countries necessarily either efficient or appropriate for the United States. "Failure" to achieve a zero rate of growth in real cost—to achieve a rate equal to the growth of gross national product (GNP), which would keep health care's share of GNP constant—or to achieve a rate as low as that achieved by a regulated system in some other country is not necessarily a deficiency. The appropriate objective is the right rate of growth in cost. That rate, in turn, depends in large part on the value that informed consumers, with both a quality and a cost stake in their decision, attach to new technology and to the use of health services. If a costly new technology is valuable in relieving pain or in reducing morbidity or mortality, a high rate of growth in cost—and the rising fraction of GNP that may result—is cause for cheer, not concern. The added cost reflects the greater benefits of higher quality. Whether rising expenditures are desirable depends on a comparison of value to cost. It is not appropriate to debate health reform within the limited framework of whether a proposal will hold cost increases to the rate of change in the GNP. The correct focus is on how to achieve a system that enables—and requires—consumers to balance value and cost as they do in other sectors.

3

Under proper incentives, a choice by informed consumers to spend more on health care and health insurance (including administration) and less on other goods and services is not to be decried.

Equity has a less precise meaning; neither economics nor logic can prove that one person's definition of fairness is necessarily superior to that of another. It is generally agreed, however, that horizontal equity is desirable: persons with the same real incomes should be treated equally. A person should not be able to pay lower taxes simply because his employer pays his health insurance premiums. It is also generally agreed that any income redistribution through the tax system should be made from those with higher incomes to those with less—vertical equity. But precisely how tax rates should rise and public benefits should decrease as real income increases is more debatable. We believe our current mildly progressive tax structure and highly progressive distribution of government welfare and transfer benefits should be maintained and that the current regressive system of tax subsidies to health insurance is an anomaly to be corrected.

3

Proposed Plan for National Health Insurance

To improve the efficiency and equity of the American health care system, we propose a plan that would guarantee coverage for all without unnecessary and unfair cross-subsidization, increase the efficiency of health care delivery and thus make more health care benefits available to more Americans, and provide the flexibility and freedom necessary to stimulate technological and administrative innovation. The plan we propose properly recognizes both the responsibilities of citizens to have adequate health insurance and the need of some for financial assistance to obtain this insurance. Our plan enhances and makes use of competitive markets; it avoids relying on the public tax and expenditure system whenever possible, to minimize tax-side distortions and to recognize the current constraints on government budgets. Our approach would permit informed individual preferences to determine the allocation of resources to health care, it would encourage the development of innovative and efficient forms of delivery, and it would advance the vitality and quality of the health care system. We call this plan Responsible National Health Insurance.

Underlying Assumptions

Our plan is based on eight assumptions.

1. Every person should be able to obtain health care on a timely and systematic basis. Society currently provides care to many of the low-income and privately uninsured families through a haphazard combination of uncompensated care, public insurance and programs, and public subsidies to some providers. It would be more effective and humane for recipients

5

and less costly for society if assistance came in the form of affordable insurance for all, rather than as grudging payment for care, often provided in the late stages of illness.

2. A monolithic, government-run or government-sponsored-and-controlled system is not necessary to provide universal health insurance. Such insurance can and should be effected instead through competitive markets, with government intervention only to make markets work and to give financial assistance to those who need it.

3. All citizens should be required to obtain a basic level of health insurance. Lack of health insurance imposes a risk that the individual will delay medical care, impairing his health and increasing costs for the rest of society, which then pays for his delayed care. Those who obtain insurance, usually by taking a job that comes with health insurance benefits in lieu of cash wages, subsidize those who remain uninsured, whether by choice or not. They receive lower cash wages to obtain insurance; the cost of that insurance and the taxes they pay are increased by the amount spent for the uninsured. Permitting individuals to remain uninsured results in inefficient use of medical care, inequity in the incidence of costs of uncompensated care, and tax-related distortions for the public subsidies they do receive. The risk of an individual's shifting costs to others has led many states to mandate that all drivers have liability insurance. The same logic applies to health insurance.

4. The ultimate obligation to obtain basic health insurance should be placed on the individual, not on the employer. This approach achieves universal coverage while satisfying individual preferences. It avoids interference with labor markets and employment contracts; it facilitates portability of coverage, employment mobility, and a competitive market; and it ensures coverage even when a person is not employed. An individual could take a job that does not carry health insurance, provided that he otherwise obtains the minimum level of insurance. Employment-based insurance is not necessarily the lowest-cost way to cover employees of small firms, which do not enjoy the scale economies of large groups; it can lead to excessive uniformity within a firm and to potential inequity. It also offers the misleading appearance that the employer pays for the insurance, whereas employees actually bear the cost by receiving lower money wages.

Placing the obligation to obtain coverage on the individual does not limit the freedom of employers or unions to offer group coverage as a fringe benefit to their employees, if they desire. Indeed, the great majority of the population would probably continue to obtain insurance through employment. There are substantial administrative cost advantages of employment-related group insurance in large firms. Moreover, group insurance may serve as a vehicle for helping individuals screen and choose among a variety of health plans; employee benefits managers develop specialized knowledge and have strong incentives to act as efficient agents for employees.

5. Government tax policy toward health insurance should be directed at making adequate insurance affordable for all, with minimum tax cost to the U.S. Treasury and minimum distortion in the choices made by individuals. This objective can best be met by requiring individuals to obtain appropriate coverage, while using predetermined tax credits, calculated on the basis of need, to achieve the desired degree of affordability, and equity. These tax credits would reduce income taxes and would be "refundable" in the sense that, if the credit exceeded an individual's tax liability, the excess would be refunded to the individual.

This assistance mechanism would replace the current system, which treats employer payments for health insurance as tax-exempt income to employees, without limit and without regard to need. The current system is horizontally inequitable, since only the employed are eligible for this tax subsidy. It is vertically inequitable, since the subsidy is higher for high-income individuals and for those who buy more comprehensive insurance. And it is contrary to the public interest; by permitting the purchase of insurance with pretax dollars, it encourages people to buy more insurance than they would otherwise purchase, thus fueling health care inflation. Because of the structure of the current tax subsidy, health care costs that an employee could pay out of pocket are covered by insurance, thus shifting a substantial proportion of the cost (equal to the individual's marginal tax bracket) to the government and hence to other taxpayers, some of whom do not have employer-paid insurance and consequently do not benefit from the same subsidy.

To extend the current tax treatment of insurance to subsidize almost everyone's purchase of insurance, as some have proposed, would perpetuate and worsen the present inequities and inefficiencies; it would also add to the already tremendous drain on the tax system (estimated at $60 billion in fiscal 1991), the real cost of which is the additional incentive distortion created by raising marginal tax rates to replace the tax revenues forgone by the tax exclusion for health insurance.

6. The required minimum level of insurance protection should be based on a family's income. Higher deductibles and out-of-pocket limits should be permitted for persons with higher incomes because they can absorb

7

more medical costs without risk of underusing care or generating bad debts. Allowing higher-income individuals to pay a larger percentage out of pocket would benefit everyone, since paying for care out of pocket results in more cost-conscious use, which in turn creates incentives for providers to keep fees and costs down. Individuals could, if they wished, purchase more complete coverage than the minimum required for their income, provided that they paid the cost of the additional coverage without government subsidy.[2]

7. Some modest increase in taxes may be needed to pay for the proposed expansion of coverage and tax credits. The amount would depend on choices about the level of required coverage and generosity of the structure of tax credits, in particular on the political will to cut back the current tax subsidies to middle- and high-income individuals. Our proposal relies on a visible and equitable source of financing in contrast with the hidden and inequitable system of financing that would result from mandating employer-paid coverage, as we discuss below.

Our proposal also contrasts with the present unfair and inefficient system. Now the amount of government assistance to those with employer-paid insurance is determined not by explicit government decision but by the amount and cost of insurance purchased and under which care for the uninsured and Medicaid beneficiaries is financed in part by a de facto excise tax on hospital charges paid by the privately insured, without regard to ability to pay.

8. A vigorous, competitive market in insurance and in health care delivery is more likely to create efficiency and high quality in health care and health insurance than is a system with one monopoly insurer operated or controlled by government. A market system, improved by purging open-ended subsidies, free riding, and cost shifting, is the most appropriate way to determine the allocation of resources to health care. A more efficient system would permit us to produce more real health benefits or more of other goods and services within our given resources. Placing the obligation to obtain insurance on the consumer would achieve universal coverage without distorting labor markets; it would encourage cost-conscious choices and a competitive market in which individuals (and employers on their behalf) have an economic interest in the selection of their insurance.

Elements of the Plan

Based on these assumptions, our plan addresses the problems of health care access and cost in the United States in the following way:

• It requires each citizen to obtain at least minimum adequate coverage against catastrophic medical expenses; because the costs that would be catastrophic necessarily depend on a family's income or wealth, the required coverage increases as family income declines. Poor people would have virtually complete coverage, and the well-to-do would not be required to buy more than basic protection that limits catastrophic out-of-pocket payments.

• The required coverage is made affordable by providing, to those families who need them, refundable fixed-dollar tax credits or adjustments in total federal taxes that are highest for those with the lowest incomes and decline at high income levels. Very poor families would receive a subsidy equal to the cost of coverage.

• The requirement to obtain coverage would be enforced through existing tax and welfare systems. The federal tax system would be used to collect the net premium (premium net of tax credit) for those persons who did not purchase insurance on their own. These premiums would be used to pay in full for coverage to be provided by private but federally or state contracted "fallback" insurers furnishing the minimum coverage for each income level.

• This system of tax credits would replace the tax treatment of health insurance, which subsidizes health insurance at the federal and state level by excluding from taxable income the health insurance premiums paid by employers. In our plan, such employer payments would be included in income subject to income tax and payroll tax.

These four features describe the qualitative nature of the basic plan. Any change in national health policy will require new administrative structures and additional payments by some citizens, and our plan is no exception. In what follows we will discuss in detail how the administrative and financing questions might be best addressed. We have no delusions of perfection in this process; there will have to be compromises among the goals of equity, efficiency, administrative simplicity, and political transparency. Many of our procedural and administrative suggestions are just suggestions and could be modified as part of the political process, based on experience gained in the transition stage. The purpose of providing detail is to show that what we propose is not only conceptually the best among imperfect alternatives but also practically feasible and that many apparent problems with the operation of this plan can be overcome.

9

4

Characteristics of Our Plan

Every person is required to obtain basic coverage, through either an individual or a family insurance plan. To satisfy this obligation and to be eligible for the tax credit, an individual must obtain coverage for specified health services; these should include basic acute care services and preventive services that are cost effective and beneficial.

Mandatory Catastrophic Coverage of Basic Services

The minimum services that must be covered are the same for everyone; plans could, however, offer more generous benefits or supplemental policies. The maximum amount of out-of-pocket expense (stop-loss) permitted is geared to income, with lower maximums required for lower-income people, to ensure that they do not face the risk of catastrophic out-of-pocket expenses, given their income.[3] A person would not satisfy his obligation if he obtained a plan with deductibles and copayments in excess of the income-related levels specified by the federal government. An individual could, if he wished, obtain coverage with lower required out-of-pocket expenses. All plans are also required to provide out-of-area coverage in emergency situations and to comply with possible requirements concerning selection, which are discussed below in connection with preferred-risk selection. The basic legislation would need to specify the core services, the conditions under which supplementation can occur, the extent of coverage, and the form of fallback coverage.

Core Services. National health insurance proposals require a definition of covered core services. Under public monopoly insurance, core services define what the government provides; under an employer or individual mandate, core services define the minimum list of services that must be covered by the mandated insurance.

The determination of core services will depend on the objectives for requiring insurance. One objective might be an intent to correct consumer misperceptions about the likelihood of incurring medical costs and the need for insurance. Another objective could be to encourage the use of care that individuals would not choose on their own but that will benefit others with altruistic concerns.

The first rationale arises from a belief that people may not recognize their risk of needing health care nor the cost that may be entailed should they become ill; they thus fail to obtain insurance. This is an often-cited reason for the high proportion of young adults who are uninsured. (Such myopia is often given as a rationale for compulsory social security.) Such poorly informed individuals may also underestimate the benefits of certain medical services. This behavior may therefore result in a lower demand for insurance and for some cost-justified services, such as preventive care with longer-term payoffs. There is little empirical evidence of such myopia, and good reason to expect that it may not be extensive. Since insurers are in business to sell insurance, it is not clear why they would not inform such potential purchasers of the value of insurance. If anything, one might fear an overselling, not underfunding. Some individuals, however, may be truly risk loving, while others may expect (usually correctly) that they will receive some care when they are severely ill, even if they cannot or will not pay. These free-riding individuals impose an external cost on others when they become ill and shift the costs of their care to others. They should be required to finance their care by obtaining the minimally required health insurance. If these misperceptions and free riding were the rationale for mandating coverage, the definition of core services would be based on the amount of insurance coverage typical persons would be willing to purchase if they had properly evaluated their risks and the benefits of medical services and insurance.

The second rationale for mandating insurance that suggests a second criterion for defining the minimum core benefits is based on the fact that medical care is a service whose use is of concern to others in the community; there are "altruistic consumption externalities." If the nonpoor want the poor to have more coverage and more use of services than the poor would obtain on their own, the nonpoor must pay for this change. This is one rationale for the tax credit or subsidy that is a key component of our plan. The fact that the United States and all other developed societies attempt to ensure some minimum access to medical care for those who cannot afford

11

to pay for themselves is strong evidence of a widespread demand for a minimum level of health care as an altruistic good.

This altruistic good rationale implies that core medical services should include all those that we as a society would be unwilling to deny others in need. This set may well differ from (and may be less than) what a typical middle-class person would choose for himself. Core services should then be defined to include all those that the taxpayers would be willing to pay for or partially subsidize for all.

As a practical matter, we assume, as we describe in the next section, that services for the poorest members of society will be fully subsidized and that subsidies will then decline and phase out at higher income levels. Accordingly, core services should be defined to include those that most taxpayers would be willing to subsidize for all, given the structure of financing.[4] Whether income taxes or some other tax base ought to be used depends, in theory, on which base is best attuned to variations in willingness to pay. In practice, we will probably have to use the roughly income-related federal income tax. Since social willingness to pay for others is likely to be more limited than private willingness to pay for one's own coverage, it seems reasonable to aim at defining the core services as the minimum required for everyone, based on social willingness to pay for those individuals who cannot afford to pay for themselves.

The definition of an ideal core set of services is primarily an exercise in exclusion. Services that are utterly useless or always harmful would be excluded. Most medical services, however, may sometimes offer both net positive health benefits and financial risk and therefore would *sometimes* be candidates for insurance coverage. Excluding services entirely from coverage is the bluntest of instruments; there are surely better ways to limit use to appropriate levels. We therefore generally prefer an inclusive definition of services that must be covered to some extent but rely on the proportion of costs covered, the circumstances in which benefits will be paid, and managed-care incentives to control excessive use.

In practice, the list of core services can be specified only by the political process, in which the interests of those who will be net recipients of benefits are balanced against those who will be net payers for those benefits. The lawmakers may decide to specify the benefits with some precision, or they may try to avoid disputes by stating the requirements in general terms and leaving the decision to other, less visible and less political forums. In either event, however, there will be disputes about the required coverage; if Congress provides a specific list of required benefits,

12

there will still be issues of interpretation, aggravated by changing medical technology. Even if it is clear that an illness is covered, it is not clear what modalities of treatment are covered.

As an initially practical solution, we advocate a definition based on the services covered by a low-cost managed-care plan that has achieved a significant market share. Expanding the core services covered under RNHI requires either higher credits or higher premium payments by citizens. Under RNHI, in contrast to other proposals for health reform, taxpayers and citizens face the full marginal cost of more generous coverage. This factor should help control a tendency toward excessively generous coverage. The core services for which coverage is mandatory are only a minimum. No one is precluded from purchasing coverage of more comprehensive services; however, public funds do not subsidize these purchases.

Income-related Coverage. Our objective is to set the minimum required coverage at a level consistent with the proper purpose of insurance—namely, spreading the financial risk of events that are beyond the economic capacity of a particular family. Insurance should be encouraged for major expenses; first-dollar coverage of routine expenses for people who can afford to make copayments should not be encouraged. Since financial capacity is defined by the size of a family's aggregate medical bills relative to its income or wealth, we propose that the minimum required coverage vary with income. No copayment would be permitted at the lowest income levels, but sizable copayments would be permitted at higher incomes. Even for those with higher incomes, however, families would be required to have coverage against truly catastrophic financial events.

Varying the required coverage with income achieves several objectives. It ensures that the family has an adequate amount left over after paying for its health care. It also ensures that families are not required to buy coverage that is of little value to them but that consumes resources to pay for insurer administration and encourages the use of medical services that are worth less than their cost. For higher incomes, substantial deductibles or copayments would be appropriate. Many high-income households might want to buy more coverage than the required minimum. The minimum is selected, though, to reduce the risk that a family would be unable to pay its bills while allowing less risk-averse families to buy insurance with moderate deductibles in order to hold down their premiums.

13

Varying the level of coverage with income produces another benefit. If low-income families have a generous subsidy for coverage, the possibility that they will underconsume care is diminished. Greater out-of-pocket payments encourage higher-income families to economize. Although research on the subject is not definitive, it appears that there may be a modestly positive relationship between income and the level of use of medical care for people with the same insurance coverage and health status. If income does affect the level of use, it follows that providing uniform coverage with uniform cost sharing would reproduce the pattern in which the rich use more. In contrast, if all expenses are fully covered by insurance, we know that the use of higher-cost care of little medical benefit would be stimulated. If we seek to make medical care use more equal (at least by bringing up the lowest level of use), insurance coverage will need to be unequal. That is, insurance coverage that increases as income falls offsets the natural tendency of use and access to decline as income falls.

Finally, tying government assistance to income enables the poor to obtain the needed insurance and provides greater equity (although a political judgment would define the extent of that equity). Since income will need to be measured to award a credit in any case, there is little additional administrative cost to designing a plan in which coverage varies with income.

Fallback Coverage Negotiated by the Government

Although most people would be expected to obtain at least the minimum coverage in a timely fashion, particularly after one or two years of experience with the system, some individuals might, nevertheless, simply fail to obtain coverage. We therefore propose that a fallback insurer be established in each geographic market area. The government would solicit bids from insurers in each area to act as fallback insurers, offering one or more plans to provide the required minimum coverage. The bids would specify the premiums that would be charged for each rating category and for each level of maximum permitted out-of-pocket expenditures. The fallback plans could involve health maintenance organizations or managed care if such plans were able to offer a low bid. Consumers might be given a choice of fallback insurer, and both a conventional insurance and a managed-care option might be offered. The government would have to designate at least one insurer to serve as fallback insurer in each area and would thus have to accept whatever premium bid was necessary to do so.

14

In return for the franchise, the fallback insurer would agree to provide coverage for every applicant.

The fallback insurer would be expected to provide coverage in two situations. Some individuals might choose to obtain coverage from this insurer rather than from other private insurers; after all, the fallback insurer would provide government-approved reasonable insurance coverage at a reasonable premium. Those individuals who fail to choose an insurer would automatically be placed with the fallback insurer; their premiums would be collected through the federal tax system and through the welfare system. The very tiny minority who pay no federal income or payroll taxes and who receive no federal transfers would be enrolled by providers with the fallback insurer when they obtained care.

The process of determining benefits and specifications for the basic package is the same process as state governments must now go through to specify what their Medicaid plans will be. Offering the package for private bidding duplicates the process now used by some states (for instance, Arizona). There is no government regulation of premiums, only a decision by government of which bids it will accept for a small minority of the population. As is well known, competitive bidding processes (given a clear specification of the product being purchased) replicate the results of ideal competitive markets.[5] The winning bid for the basic plan for people below the poverty line then sets the amount of the maximum tax credit.

Since the government must specify coverage and obtain bids for the fallback insurer, especially for low-income persons, there is no way to avoid some government involvement in this sector. We believe that the approach we have described keeps the extent of government interference in the choices people make to the minimum. The government does not specify prices paid to providers, methods of cost containment, or providers to be included in a plan. Its only role is to provide a credit and make sure that people select plans that meet minimum guidelines. While no policy design can prevent politicians or bureaucrats with a taste for regulation and control from trying to meddle, the design we have suggested keeps opportunities for doing so to a minimum.

In a similar fashion, limiting the amount of the credit at any income to the amount needed so that the family can afford the required coverage and setting the required coverage as a minimum that declines with increasing income minimize the extent to which the government uses funds under its control to finance insurance and medical care.

Universal Tax Credits or Vouchers

Employer payments for health insurance premiums are currently tax-exempt compensation to employees. This exemption distorts insurance markets and offers larger tax subsidies to higher-income people. Our plan would eliminate the exclusion, replacing it with a system of refundable tax credits (which are in essence vouchers for persons with little or no tax liability) inversely related to a family's income. Very low income individuals would be entitled to a tax credit or voucher at least sufficient to cover the cost of the basic but comprehensive insurance policy with zero or minimal copayments. As incomes rise from the low cutoff level, the credit will fall below the cost of the policy, and the person will have to pay part of the policy premium as well as the out-of-pocket payments.

The "full cost" credit for the poor would depend on the cost of obtaining the required coverage. So that the lowest-income families can afford coverage, it may be necessary to tie the full cost credit they receive to the negotiated premium for fallback coverage. The credit also could be adjusted to reflect each individual's or family's actuarial category (age, gender, and family size) or its particular risk, depending on the design option selected to mitigate the effects of risk variation discussed below.

One policy issue is whether credits should vary across different geographic areas. If the tax credit at any income level were uniform—calculated, for instance, on a national average of insurance costs—people of a given income living in lower-cost areas who pay less for insurance would have more income left over to spend on other things.

Whether there should be a national rate (after a transition period) is a matter of policy design best left to Congress and the political process. The resolution will depend on perceptions of the reasons for the cost differentials between regions, particularly whether the differential is based upon unavoidable differences in medical costs, inefficient production or inappropriate use of health care resources, or differences in the quality of care.[6]

A similar question of whether area differences in health care costs should be reflected in the amount of federal assistance has arisen in connection with the Diagnostic Related Group (DRG) rates under the Medicare Prospective Payment System (PPS). The original differential in rates between urban and rural hospitals, which was based on the belief that there are valid differences in cost, is being phased out; but the rates may still vary between urban and rural hospitals as the standardized rate is adjusted by particular identified cost differentials such as wages and case mix. The decision is far more limiting under PPS than it would be under RNHI; the DRG rate set by the government constitutes the full amount of the hospital's reimbursement for treating a Medicare patient; the hospital cannot bill the patient for the difference. Under RNHI, however, except for the poorest individual who cannot and is not expected to supplement the government contribution, the tax credit does not have to be a perfect reflection of the cost of insurance. The federal tax credit is by definition an assistance to the individual to purchase insurance; the individual is expected to make his own contribution to the purchase of insurance. The government tax credit, unlike the DRG rate, does not set the price for the insurance.

We propose to replace the current exclusion of employment-related premiums from taxation with a fixed-dollar or closed-end tax credit because it is a way of improving both equity and efficiency. The current tax treatment of health insurance is horizontally inequitable because it depends on employment status and employer contribution. It is vertically inequitable because the subsidy per dollar of insurance premium is greater for persons paying higher marginal income and payroll tax rates. An open-ended tax exclusion implies larger subsidies for high-income workers and those who choose more generous coverage. Our plan would treat any employer premium payments (and premiums employees pay out of flexible benefit accounts) as part of taxable compensation, to be reported on the employee's W-2 form. Tax credits toward the purchase of the obligatory coverage would be provided to all, based on income, regardless of how the insurance is obtained.

The fundamental reason for the change is simple: "employer-paid" health insurance is part of compensation and should therefore be included in taxable compensation. The tax credit is then determined by the person's total income, without regard to the division between total income, wage income, and health insurance premiums. In the most fundamental sense, our proposed tax credits adjust the progressivity of the income tax, making it modestly more progressive. This modest increase in progressivity might be justified on the grounds that requiring purchase of insurance is, in itself, like a regressive tax (though one that the great majority of lower-income persons—who already have insurance—currently pay). The higher income-related credits offset this regressive payment.

Such a closed-end tax credit also gives proper incentives for efficiency. The amount of the credit is fixed for any family; it is based on the family's income, and the actuarial factors discussed below, and perhaps the cost of insurance in its geographic area. The credit is not calculated on the basis of the amount the family actually spends on health care or health insurance; buying more lavish insurance or using more medical care does not increase the amount of the credit received. A *fixed* tax credit does not distort incentives about how much insurance to buy, what type of insurance to buy, or where to buy that insurance. In contrast, because the amount of tax avoided grows as the current tax exclusion grows, the exclusion encourages the purchase of overly lavish and underaggressive health insurance.

The use of a tax credit of predetermined value, rather than one that is some proportion of the premium cost of the insurance policy the family chooses to buy, is a critical feature that makes our plan more efficient and less intrusive than that proposed by the Heritage Foundation. Not only is a fixed credit less distortive of the type or amount of insurance purchased than is such a variable credit, but it is much easier to administer—since the tax credit can generally be calculated without knowing what a person actually paid for insurance or medical care: we need to know only the person's income.[7] Combining a fixed tax credit with a requirement to buy insurance means that the credit does not change the individual's incentives; the credit only eases the financial consequences of the requirement to buy insurance.

Treatment of "Employer-paid" Group Insurance Premiums. While individuals will satisfy the requirement to buy coverage in various ways, we suspect that the great majority will continue to obtain their insurance in connection with employment, although we do anticipate that other groups, such as banks, schools, and credit unions or even insurance brokers and agents could become intermediaries for obtaining insurance, once the current tax bias in favor of the employment setting is eliminated.

Many employers will continue to contribute to employee insurance premiums. Since the employer's contribution is taxable income, the question is how this contribution should be distributed across workers. The most appropriate administrative structure is probably one in which the employer is free to designate how much of a total premium paid for group insurance is to be attributed to each employee; the only constraint is that the employer must allocate the entire group premium among employees if it is to be treated as employee compensation and therefore as an expense of doing business.

In the simplest case, in which the employer makes a fixed-dollar payment for all employees and then has them pay any additional premium, the administrative calculation would be easy: this fixed-dollar amount would be added to each employee's reported wage income. If all workers are of the same risk and the employer "paid" the entire net premium, it would likewise be obvious that the same dollar amount should be attributed to each worker and added to taxable compensation.[8]

But what happens if workers have somewhat different risk levels (for example, because of age) but the employer pays a single premium, as is the case for self-insured firms and large group purchasers? In this case, the most sensible strategy would be to permit the employer (or the union or employee group) to choose how it wishes to allocate the total premium expense across employees. Indirectly, the allocation method would be constrained by competition in the labor market, since workers evaluate job options on the basis of both money and fringe benefits. Our plan leaves it up to the employer or union to decide how to deal with differences among employees, such as family size and composition, when this is not determined by an insurer's premium calculation.

There is one potential complication. Suppose the employer or union does not vary the reported premium contribution for a group of workers who have the same skill level and cash wages but differ in expected health benefits because of differences in age or health status. By reporting a premium contribution that does not vary with employee risk class, the employer understates full compensation of higher-risk workers and overstates compensation of lower-risk workers. Here again there is a trade-off between administrative complexity and equity. Technically the premium attributable to a worker should be based on that worker's expected benefit, but ascertaining this would be extraordinarily complex. The amount of unfairness involved seems small relative to the administrative cost, since the only impact is a slight adjustment in taxable income.

Note that, with these adjustments, there would be subtle changes in the income categories of different individuals. Consider two workers who both currently receive $20,000 in money income, but one also gets a health insurance policy worth $2,000. Our plan would not classify these individuals in the same money income category, since the "before premium" income of the two workers would be $20,000 and $22,000, respectively. Since these individuals do not have equal consumption opportunities, it is appropriate to tax them differently, and that is what our plan would do. The person who formerly had to buy his own insurance policy would pay payroll and income taxes (if any) on an income of $20,000 and receive the tax credit appropriate to an income of $20,000. In contrast, the person who received health insurance as a fringe benefit would pay the taxes and receive the credits appropriate for an income of $22,000. This second employee would be regarded as a higher-cost employee in any labor market, and, if his skills justified receipt of total compensation worth $22,000, he should pay tax on that compensation.

Financial Impact. The net effect of RNHI on the after-tax cost of health insurance will differ across families, depending on their incomes and on the level of the tax credits adopted. In general, lower-income persons who currently obtain either individual or employment-based group insurance will enjoy a net reduction in taxes, since their tax credit under the proposal would probably exceed the value to them of the current tax exclusion. Indeed, at incomes below the poverty line, the tax credit would equal the premium; the insurance would be wholly financed by the government.

Higher-income employees, who benefit most from the current tax loophole, would pay higher taxes on balance; this would be an important revenue source for financing the new subsidies to the low-income families. The tax credit will phase out at zero for sufficiently high incomes; at the same time, the required level of coverage and hence the premium for the mandated plan would also decline with income, but expected out-of-pocket costs for those who buy only the minimum coverage would increase. On balance high-income families would pay a larger fraction of the cost of their health care than at present. Of course, over time the elimination of the tax loophole will increase efficiency and probably slow the rate of growth in health care costs, so that the real cost of health care may be lower than under the status quo even for higher-income families.

Setting the income threshold for eligibility for a full cost credit and the subsequent phasing down of credits and required coverage are basically political decisions. These decisions, together with the number of persons at each income level and the definition of core services, will determine the fiscal cost of the program. These choices will presumably depend on balancing the political cost of increasing taxes with the political gain of providing more generous subsidies and will be adjusted over time if the program proves to be more (or less) expensive than anticipated. Operationally, the size of the subsidy required to make the basic benefits package available to those with low incomes would be determined by the cost to insurers of providing the basic benefits, because the government would be required to pay enough to cover the cost of at least one fallback insurer in each area.

RNHI has a very strong advantage in encouraging rational democratic political choice—an advantage to voters, though not necessarily to politicians. The level and distribution of subsidies required, and the determination of who will be taxed to provide them, will be visible to voters as well as to legislators. It will be less possible than it is now for the political process to hide subsidies to middle- and high-income groups, while financing those benefits with regressive taxes. The trade-offs between beneficiaries and taxpayers will be obvious and subject to discussion and will likely be decided in open political debate. If the cost of subsidies increases over time, we would expect that Congress would consider the basic benefits package, the size of the subsidy in relation to different income groups, the necessary federal appropriations, and the required taxes. We would avoid useless and misleading discussions about "needed" care and about "giving" benefits, without facing up to the question of who will pay for them.

5

How the Program Would Operate

Employed Individuals and Their Families

Under RNHI, any arrangement between the individual and the employer for payment of premium and choice of coverage beyond the minimum would be left to employment negotiations, either individually or collectively bargained. The employer might "pay" the premium by reducing wages by the cost of coverage. In this case, the employer's contribution would be part of the taxable income to the employee. Alternatively, the employee might be explicitly responsible for payment to the group insurer, either directly or through a checkoff from the paycheck. The employer would report the type of coverage the employee obtains and payments the employer makes (if any) on the employee's W-2 form. The individual would receive the tax credit, calculated on his income inclusive of any employer-paid premiums.

Since premiums that the employer pays on behalf of the employee would be included in employees' taxable income, our plan avoids irrelevant questions like, Should the credit depend on what the employee pays or what the employer pays, or their sum? In our approach, the answer is, None of the above. The credit depends only on the total income paid to the employee, not on the division of an employer's contribution between wages and insurance benefits.

If the employer did not arrange a health plan that met the obligatory standards, all employees would be required to present evidence that they had obtained the additional coverage as part of filling out the W-4 form to determine federal income tax withholding from wages; this would reflect the credit to which they are entitled. If no evidence of coverage were provided, an additional amount to pay the premium for fallback insurance would be withheld from the paycheck, along with the conventional withholding for federal income tax purposes. Individuals would then be covered automatically by the fallback insurer, and the amount withheld would go toward the fallback insurance premiums. The net amount withheld would depend, of course, on both the premium negotiated by the government with the fallback insurer and on the amount of the individual's tax credit.

At the end of the tax year, when family income is known with certainty, the tax credit would be adjusted. In multiple-worker families, only one family member would need to obtain coverage for the family, and the size of the credit would depend on the size of the family income.

The Self-employed

The self-employed have been allowed to deduct 25 percent of any health insurance premiums (in contrast to the 100 percent deduction for employer payments on behalf of employees). This deduction for the self-employed would also be replaced by the universal system of income-related tax credits. The self-employed would be required to obtain coverage but could adjust their estimated federal income tax payments to reflect the expected credit due. If they failed to obtain private insurance coverage, they would be required to include their expected net premium payment (for the fallback insurance) in their prepayment of estimated taxes. Failure to pay this premium as part of one's estimated tax would be subject to the same penalties as are now applied for underpayment of estimated taxes.

Persons Who Are Not Employed

Dependents in families in which at least one person is employed could be covered through a family plan of an employed family member, or the family might choose to obtain coverage in some other group. Persons in families receiving welfare or transfer payments from the government either would use their voucher or would be covered by the fallback insurer. Persons in families without either an employed person or a recipient of federal transfer payments would also be required to obtain coverage. There are very few such persons, and most of them would be eligible for the 100 percent subsidy.

Individuals with incomes (for example, from property or securities) large enough to have positive tax liabilities could reduce their payment of estimated taxes to reflect the expected tax credit for insurance premiums. They would be required to include as part of their estimated tax expected

23

net premium payment for fallback insurance if they could not show proof of purchase of private insurance.

Low Income

Persons whose incomes were too low to have a tax liability could purchase coverage and file to receive the refundable credit. Many low-income individuals, however, could not afford to pay the monthly premium cost out of pocket, even if they were entitled to a full refund at the end of the tax year. The administrative machinery of welfare could be used to bridge this gap. The local welfare agency would verify income status, collect the net premium payment due from the individual (if any), and issue the individual a voucher or advance for the cost of coverage, to be used to enroll either in a private plan meeting the obligatory standards or in the fallback plan. The welfare agency would receive the tax credit due to the individual.

If such an individual received government cash assistance, any net premium contribution due could be withheld from his cash payments. Using local welfare agencies to verify income and issue a voucher draws on a bureaucracy that is already set up to verify income status and would facilitate prompt enrollment of poor individuals who could not afford or simply failed to obtain coverage on their own. If there were no private plan that the individual could purchase with his credit, he could be covered by the fallback carrier. His credit would then be paid to the fallback insurer; the level of the credit (adjusted for risk, as described below) is defined to be sufficient to cover the cost of fallback insurance for low-income people.

Variations in Income

Families are subject to unexpected variations in their incomes over time. As noted, preliminary determinations of the tax credit and the required coverage could be based on an estimate of the family's income. When the family's total income is known at the end of the year, any necessary adjustments in the tax credits could be made. The maximum permitted out-of-pocket payment in the family's insurance policy would, in an ideal situation, also change if income changed.

Administrative complexity associated with such changes could be kept down by defining required coverage for intervals of income, so that fluctuations in income would rarely change the required minimum coverage. Moreover, a decline in income would not cause a problem for the many families who would buy more than the minimum coverage. For those few families who do experience a major unexpected drop in income and have expenses so high that they exceed the maximum out-of-pocket expenses for the lower-income level, the simplest solution would be to require the insurance plan to cover more out-of-pocket payments and receive the increased credit at the end of the year to pay the higher premium.

Effect on Medicaid

The acute-care coverage provided by Medicaid to persons under age sixty-five would be replaced by the proposed system. Individuals would be eligible for the credit based on their income, regardless of their categorical status. Almost all persons now eligible for Medicaid would be eligible for a subsidy equal to the full cost of minimum coverage.

A distinct advantage of our plan is that it would eliminate the notch disincentive now faced by Medicaid eligibles who lose their subsidized health coverage completely as soon as they earn income sufficient to raise them above the eligibility threshold. Under the current Medicaid system, anyone who increases his earnings during the year and exceeds the Medicaid eligibility standard loses insurance coverage unless he works for an employer who provides coverage. Our plan would ensure continued coverage for the individual even as income changed during the year. The variations among state Medicaid programs and the different amounts contributed by the states to Medicaid beneficiaries would be ended. A similarly situated individual would receive the same coverage, regardless of the state in which he lived. States, like employers, could, if they wished, provide supplemental assistance in addition to the federal contribution, but all individuals would be covered by the national minimum standard of coverage.

If no adjustments were made, full federal financing of RNHI would relieve the states of their expenditure burden in proportion to the amount they currently devote to the non-elderly acute-care portion of their Medicaid programs. A number of options are available to Congress to preserve some state contributions. A "maintenance-of-effort" rule could require states to continue their present contributions by making payments to the federal government, thus maintaining the current disparities in state expenditures for Medicaid. It could phase out any maintenance-of-effort requirement until no state was making any contribution, or it could phase in a requirement that resulted in all states paying the same proportion of income.

Congress's response to these options and the extent to which it requires states to contribute to the health care of their citizens depend upon broader issues of federalism and political balance. Our proposal operates regardless of how Congress and the states resolve their respective roles.

At the same time, RNHI ensures that the level of care and the amount the federal government provides for assistance in obtaining coverage are addressed explicitly and jointly. Under the current Medicaid matching process, the financial obligation of the federal government is determined for it by the states without its participation or consent, since the states administer the Medicaid program. At the same time, states have been forced to contribute resources based on additional requirements imposed by the federal government. Our proposal avoids the separation of authority from financial responsibility that occurs under the current Medicaid system.

Treatment of Medicare

Medicare can be treated under RNHI in various ways. It can be kept separate from RNHI; it can be phased into RNHI; or Medicare beneficiaries can be given the opportunity to decide voluntarily whether to participate in RNHI. Another option would be to leave current Medicare beneficiaries in that program and phase in RNHI for others as they aged into Medicare eligibility. The choice is a political decision.

Allowing a voluntary choice between Medicare and RNHI would increase the total cost of the Medicare program if all the aged were still funded from Medicare funds. For low-income aged, the income-related tax credit approach of RNHI would be preferable to current Medicare benefits, which include sizable deductibles and copayments. It is therefore likely that these Medicare beneficiaries would choose to participate in RNHI. High-income aged would probably prefer to keep their current Medicare benefits since they would likely face greater out-of-pocket payments under RNHI and since they receive a substantial subsidy from taxpayers in general (especially for Part B). The middle-income aged would have to evaluate whether their out-of-pocket payments are lower under RNHI or Medicare.

Patient Protection Measures

State-mandated benefit laws, which currently apply to commercial insurers but not to self-insured firms, would be preempted. There is little social rationale for permitting states to enact laws requiring or regulating coverage once a federal requirement for universal coverage of core benefits is in place.

In practice, these state laws often resemble special interest legislation, benefiting the providers of the mandated services but raising the cost of coverage to consumers. If states were permitted to enact such laws, the resulting increase in the cost of coverage would inevitably lead to a demand for increased federal tax credits, since credits calculated to cover the cost of basic coverage alone would be insufficient. There is no reason why federal taxpayers should finance the cost of special benefits for consumers and providers of these services in some states.

States might be permitted (though not encouraged) to regulate some aspects of coverage supplementary to the basic plan. Anticompetitive laws that restrict provider selection or utilization review should be preempted. The current unequal treatment of commercial insurers and self-insurers in financing high-risk pools would also be eliminated under our plan. A patient protection fund, administered by either the states or the federal government, would be created to compensate enrollees for benefits due in the event that a plan became insolvent during a contract period. The fund would be financed by assessments on insurers and the benefit payments of qualified self-insured firms. In the transition phase, current state and federal solvency rules would be continued. As part of the definition developed for plans that satisfy the minimum insurance requirement, some review of the solvency rules (for commercial and self-insured plans) may need to be undertaken. Finally, an independent commission would be created to evaluate the program's performance and to recommend any changes.

Supplementation

Compulsory coverage would define the minimum coverage with respect to core services covered and the maximum exposure to out-of-pocket costs. Many individuals would therefore probably choose to buy coverage with more comprehensive services or with lower out-of-pocket costs.

Such supplementation raises normative issues—should the extent of such supplementation be left totally to the free market? The argument for permitting supplementation is, of course, individual freedom to satisfy diverse consumer preferences. The arguments against total freedom to supplement are based on notions of norms, arising from jointness in production or pricing effects, and on notions of public production. We believe that these arguments do not on balance support limits on supplementation.

Jointness in Production. Purchase of supplementary insurance by some may raise norms of care and hence costs of medical care for others. This spillover can operate through joint costs in the production of medical care. Purchases of supplementary insurance by some may increase the rate of technical change, particularly change that enhances the range of relatively costly technologies available. If each technology offered entails fixed costs, the range of offerings is limited. As the fraction of the population demanding high-cost technologies increases, the costs of producing less expensive technologies may increase if demand for them falls below the minimum efficient scale. Some technologies for which there is relatively low demand will be dropped entirely. This, however, is no different from the quite general question of whether competitive markets produce the optimal range of product qualities.

Price Levels. An increase in insurance coverage, defined by copayments, generally reduces total market demand elasticity and hence raises the fees charged by providers. This applies only in the context of passive fee-for-service reimbursement and only if the number of persons insulated from prices is a large fraction of the market. Conversely, managed care and preferred provider plans will tend to increase demand elasticity.

A converse argument is that insurers have weak incentives to invest in provider-targeted strategies to control moral hazard because of spillover effects to competitors. Thus if some consumers buy supplementary coverage that, for example, does not have strict utilization review for hospitalizations or substitution of generic for brand name drugs, provider behavior patterns in general will be less cost conscious. This is simply another variant of the fixed-norms argument and does not justify limits on supplementation of insurance and medical care.

Public Production. In monopoly public systems the fundamental problem is price constraint in the form of fixed salaries or prices for professional workers, with imperfect monitoring of how their hours are spent. Not only can the public sector not raise wage rates to compete with the private sector but the services provided to the public sector for the fixed wage may actually be less than those contracted for. This situation is exacerbated if specialists manipulate queues in the public sector to maximize demand for their private sector business.

Such problems should not occur, however, in a health care system in which the required universal level of coverage is provided by competing private insurers rather than by a monopoly system. In this case, the reimbursement systems used by private insurers become one dimension of competition. Those insurers that choose to compete by offering high-cost, high-quality products will design employment and fee packages that attract the necessary supply of good physicians. Other plans will compete for market niches that offer good quality but lower-cost products, possibly with more nonprice rationing of services, as many HMOs currently do. But they will still have to pay enough to attract the required number of specialists of adequate quality. Thus a private market with demand for diversity satisfied by private offerings of stand-alone policies avoids the distortions that result when supplementation takes the form of private gap insurance added on to a budget-constrained, public provider of core services.

Societies that begin their health care systems as public monopoly insurance systems become more willing to tolerate private supplementary coverage as costs and demands for public funds push up against fiscal constraints. Supplementary coverage is an escape valve that releases some pressure on the queues for free public services. It also permits governments to raise copayments in the public system, since the argument can be made that those who want more protection can buy gap insurance. Consistent with this, supplementary insurance is permitted in the United Kingdom and New Zealand, where the public system has encountered tighter fiscal constraints. Supplementary insurance is not permitted in Canada, though, where the initial endowment of the public system was more generous and public fiscal constraints have been less binding because of more rapid growth rates and a higher starting point.

When a public monopoly system in a democratic country runs into tight fiscal constraints for a sustained period, supplementation is likely to be permitted in response to public dissatisfaction with service availability in the public system and political constraints on raising the public funds necessary to raise service levels for everyone. Once private supplementation of a public system is permitted—and this is almost inevitable in the long run—the arguments are overwhelming in favor of a system such as we propose, with competing private insurers rather than a public monopoly insurer and provider of core services with private supplementary coverage for those who want it.

With competing private insurers, consumers generally will obtain their coverage from a single insurer. Those that want to buy more than core coverage will buy a single, more comprehensive policy. This is more efficient than having one policy for core services and another separate supplementary policy, which entails higher overhead due to duplicative enrollment costs and more significant costs of coordinating coverages, as each insurer must protect against cost shifting by the other. These costs are even more severe if the insurer for core services is the government. In that case there are typically separate reimbursement systems and possibly different providers, leading to lack of coordination of care, duplication of some services, and omission of others. Since there will be private supplementation if government provides the core services, having the private insurer provide the core coverage in the first instance is more efficient.

6
Adverse and Preferred Risk Selection

Adverse selection occurs when the policyholder is better able to anticipate expenses than the insurer and then acts on that knowledge by deciding whether or not to buy coverage and how much coverage to buy. People who anticipate being high users will be likely to buy extensive coverage, while those who expect to have low use will either not buy insurance or buy policies with less coverage. Because our plan obligates individuals to buy the core coverage, adverse selection is impossible in the market for the required coverage. The obligation to buy coverage means that the most common vehicle for adverse selection, dropping coverage when one expects to be well, is not available under our plan. This critical feature distinguishes our plan from Alain Enthoven's Consumer Choice Plan,[9] in which coverage is not mandated (although it is partially subsidized) for the self-employed and persons with no labor income.

Adverse Selection

One should not, in any case, overemphasize the role of adverse selection in actual insurance markets; it affects only the minority in small group and individual markets. Our plan, however, does more: it wholly breaks the vicious circle of adverse selection. It does this by requiring that people buy basic coverage even when they expect to be good risks. Each insurer can thus expect to get a random slice of all risks, and there is no need to charge a premium higher than the average expected for a given risk class. More formally, adverse selection, defined as the phenomenon in which insurance purchasers with private knowledge buy amounts of insurance based on that knowledge, is literally impossible under our plan with regard to the basic

31

insurance. The reason is simple: all *must* buy, regardless of what they know or think they know.

To be sure, adverse selection for supplemental coverage in excess of the basic amount can still exist. Since this is optional coverage, however, it is a matter of much less social concern. Moreover, both the preservation of group insurance and the requirement of guaranteed renewability should combine to make adverse selection in these supplemental markets of minimal importance. That is, the only insurance which, in the worst case, an insurer might price very high or refuse to renew is insurance that in society's judgment is not really necessary.

Preferred Risk Selection

Incentives for preferred risk selection, or for risk rating, in contrast, might remain under our plan, depending on how insurance is priced or required to be priced. In any insurance market with more than one insurer, insurers tend to charge higher premiums to persons who they judge are high risks and lower premiums to those who they believe are low risks. At least some of this variation in premium with the level of risk is sometimes regarded as unfair.

Risk rating, permitting insurers to vary premiums by expected cost, can in principle have the beneficial effect of rewarding and therefore encouraging risk-reducing behavior, such as not smoking. But some factors that make individuals high risk are beyond their control. The phenomenon of risk rating is to be criticized primarily on equity grounds; risk rating means that higher risks will pay more than average. It may be considered politically unacceptable to have the sick pay higher costs for coverage, particularly as ill health may also have reduced their ability to work. (If they are unable to work, however, their tax credit will automatically increase as income falls.) Very high-risk individuals may be unable to obtain coverage at premiums that they can afford. Requiring insurers to charge premiums that do not reflect risk, however, does not solve the problem. Insurers will sell only to lower risks; they will engage in "cream skimming" or preferred risk selection. Clearly, a national health insurance plan that relies on private insurance markets must address these possible effects of competitive markets.

A number of different strategies might be chosen to deal with this difficult problem; they involve different trade-offs between the administrative costs of tailoring tax credits to risk and the administrative costs of trying to regulate insurers to limit the extent of risk rating. That is, there is a trade-off between the objective of maximizing the extent of competition among insurers, and the administrative cost of tailoring credits to each family's circumstances.

It is important, first of all, to keep this problem in perspective. The problem of substantially increased insurance premiums based on insurer perceptions of risk differences will affect only a small minority of families at any time. Only about 3 percent of the population report themselves to be in fair or poor health, and it is conventionally believed that the proportion of the population that is uninsurable (requiring market premiums so high as to be infeasible) is less than 1 percent of the under-sixty-five population. Moreover, risk rating by insurers depends on the distinctions in risk that insurers can economically identify, not on all true differences. Surprisingly, no research identifies the distribution of premiums that insurers, using their conventional risk rating and underwriting rules, would charge to a random slice of the population.

To be sure, current insurance markets, especially small group markets, seem to be more widely affected by substantial jumps in premiums or refusals to insure after a high-cost illness. Some of this behavior is probably traceable to fears of adverse selection: even an apparently mild case of asthma in a family, or a moderately expensive illness in a small group, triggers a substantial jump in premiums because the insurer fears that these indicators may signal a higher-cost illness known to the family or the group. As noted, such adverse selection will be ended by the requirement in our plan that all persons obtain coverage.

The fact that the problem of high risk is confined to a small minority means that one would not sacrifice much participation in a competitive insurance market even if all persons with risks substantially above average were assigned to a state-run high-risk pool. It also means that government regulation to engineer some type of transfers among risks—so-called community rating—might also have only a small effect once premiums were adjusted for obvious demographic characteristics. The relatively limited character of the problem, however, means as well that it would not be difficult to administer a small program of special risk-rated credits and to preserve the full functioning of the market. We now discuss four options for dealing with risk variation.

Individual Rating of Premiums and Credits Combined with Mandatory Guaranteed Renewability. An ideal solution would be the rating of both premiums and tax credits on the basis of risk factors. Insurers would charge people at any level of risk their expected cost of coverage, and the government would also adjust tax credits according to expected cost. If the government has the same information in setting credits as do insurers in setting premiums, this process could eliminate unintended differences in the out-of-pocket cost of coverage among individuals. The government could differentiate between those elements of increased cost that it would recognize in calculating the tax credit (such as illness) and those (for example, smoking) that it would not and adjust the credit by the estimated actuarial cost of those risk factors that it determined should be reflected in the calculation of the credit. The problem with achieving this ideal is the administrative cost and complexity of having the government determine risk levels.

Although it might be administratively difficult to achieve risk rating of credits that perfectly matches what insurers would charge, rating on the basis of age and broad illness categories is feasible. An additional strategy to reduce the administrative problem would involve requiring every person to buy coverage that provides limited-term renewability at non–risk-rated premiums for a period, with the government then adjusting credits upward only for the rarer long-term chronic illness. A second part of the strategy would permit individuals to claim tax credits larger than the standard for their income if they provided one of two kinds of evidence of need: (1) evidence of being quoted premiums designed for nonstandard risks and (2) evidence that they have a condition that would classify them as long-term high risks. Higher than average premiums alone could just reflect insurer inefficiency; that is why we do not tie the credit to actual premiums.[10] One might want to require both kinds of information if one distrusted insurer premium-rating practices.

We also envision an uninsured corridor or range in which modestly elevated premiums would still be judged affordable and therefore not requiring adjustments in credits. Permitting some premiums higher than standard—for instance, perhaps up to 50 percent higher—would also permit insurers to build in financial incentives to discourage bad health behaviors, such as smoking, by modestly surcharging premiums. If an individual can show that a number of insurers, including the fallback insurer, have required premiums in excess of 150 percent of the standard premium for the person's geographic area and age, then the person could apply for a supplemental credit as part of the regular process of determining credits. To minimize administrative costs, the credit could be a simple percentage add-on to the standard credit.

How would limited-term guaranteed renewability work? Guaranteed renewability at standard premiums means that the insurers cannot raise premiums charged to any insured or group of insureds by more than the rate of increase for a standard risk (or if there are no standard risks, the rate would be tied to an index of medical expenditures). This requirement, however, would be limited in time to perhaps three years. Thus an insurer could not raise a person's premium this year, next year, or the year after based on a change in medical condition today but could eventually risk adjust the premium. Insurance policies are conventionally written on a one-year basis; changes in the insured's risk status during that time do not change the premium. Guaranteed renewability in effect extends the period in which premiums are guaranteed (permitting upward adjustments for increases in cost in the health care sector). It has been proposed as a requirement for insurance policies by the National Association of Insurance Commissioners, although the NAIC's approach would not limit the term and would permit some limited risk adjustment.

We require limited guaranteed renewability because rational insurance purchasing requires it. Illnesses do not necessarily respect the twelve months of a year; they may start in one period and end in another. Buying a policy that permits a substantial jump in premiums is like having a fire insurance policy in which the premiums could be raised once one's house caught on fire. Illness typically proceeds at a somewhat slower pace than a fire, but the principle is the same: a risk-averse person should be protected against the risk of an increase in premiums.

We do not require unlimited or lifetime guaranteed renewability, however, because such a long guarantee is probably infeasible, would require a heavy regulatory burden, would lock individuals into particular insurers, and would not be equitable. Unlimited guaranteed renewability presents the problem of insuring against a lifetime chronic condition or illness. To collect enough premiums to cover the cost, either a substantial premium must be paid up front or the individual must be prevented from switching insurers. Both of these devices may be impossible for insurers to implement, and both have the effect of attaching an individual to a given insurer regardless of that insurer's performance. Moreover, pooling the risk of lifetime catastrophic expenses for chronic illness within small insurers or in small groups will not spread the cost over the entire community; rather, that cost will fall more heavily on those groups unlucky enough to contain disproportionate numbers of members with such illnesses.

Participation in the financing of serious and costly chronic illness is an appropriate function of government. The best way to structure this is to adjust tax credits so that they are more generous for people with chronic illness but then to permit those people to participate in the same type of competitive insurance markets as others. Such transfers will be an explicit object of political choice—financing of care for people with AIDS, for example, will require more generous tax-financed transfers to those with the condition.

Such an explicit process of designating persons at high risk for chronic illness should greatly reduce the administrative cost of risk-related credits, once RNHI is phased in. A person who develops a chronic illness that may eventually result in being rated as a high risk goes through a sequential process of designation, targeting for changes in risk category after some time, and eventual premium adjustment. Along the way, explicit designation of reasons for insurer actions can provide the information needed to trigger a higher than average tax credit. The best predictor of an individual's medical care cost next year, for example, is this year's level of expenditures. The ability of any one year's relative expenditure level to predict future expenditures, however, falls off rapidly after the first subsequent year. Since guaranteed renewability forbids raising premiums for the next two or three years for almost all persons, temporary but severe illnesses could not trigger higher premiums or higher credits. Upward adjustments in premiums and credits would be limited to persons who had experienced long periods of above-average expenditure—the small number of persons with costly and chronic illness for whom a public subsidy is appropriate in any case.

With required guaranteed renewability, the need for such risk-related credits would be limited to those with substantially elevated lifetime expected expenses from long-term chronic conditions; with guaranteed renewability, higher than average claims in one year would not be permitted to trigger either substantially higher premiums or the designation of a chronic high-risk condition for the renewal period. We would therefore anticipate that only a small fraction of citizens, surely less than 5 percent of the population at any time, would need to qualify for a risk-related supplemental credit. The administrative cost burden would therefore be small.

When coverage is arranged through group purchasing—employment-related or otherwise—providing risk-related credits does set up modest incentives for the group to charge its members higher premiums for serious chronic illnesses; the group knows that the high-cost member will recoup some of the surcharge from the government. A less than complete adjustment in the credit, however, is probably enough to limit any such risk rating within groups to the rare high-cost chronic illness. And in the case of an individual who does have such an illness, it *is* fair that the cost of assisting in financing be spread over all taxpayers, rather than just among those with whom the individual happens to work or to buy insurance. Neither the employer nor the other employees in a group (or the other members of a non–employment-related group) have a greater ethical obligation to help the high-cost individual than other citizens. For this reason, a tax-credit scheme spreads the burden in the widest and fairest way; this is to be preferred to a strategy of forcing the group to care for its own, precisely because the high risks are not *its* own.

As a practical matter, a perfect alignment of the rating of credits and premiums may not be feasible. If the information available to the government in setting credits is less complete than that used by insurers in setting premiums, higher-risk individuals within tax-credit categories would pay higher net costs for coverage. Of course, insurers may know more about the risk of an individual than the federal program that calculates the credits, but this should not be assumed to be a serious problem until there is some experience with such arrangements. As long as what the insurers know does not produce substantially higher or lower premiums than the information that the federal program uses in setting the credit, the amount of risk or inequity can be kept to a moderate level.

The severity of the after-credit variation in net premium cost among individuals is an empirical question. Both the required guaranteed renewability that we envision and the minimal underwriting standards that are required by low administrative costs in medium to large employment-based group insurance will mean that, even for most individuals at above-average risk in any period, premiums will still be affordable. Among those persons who do not buy their insurance in groups, especially in the early years of RNHI, however, some individuals will experience substantial jumps (up or down) in their premiums as their assessed risk levels change. Some transitional cushioning of such variations might be appropriate.

The fallback insurer could provide a low-cost vehicle for identifying above-average risks. To do its own risk rating, the fallback insurer will have to implement procedures for identifying those risks. Competitive bidding guarantees that the fallback insurer's premium is close to the expected cost for each class of insured, and the insurer's interest in maximizing profits ensures that cost-effective information for risk classification will be collected. Observation that the fallback insurer has charged an individual a significantly above-average premium is then sufficient indication to the government that a high-risk tax credit should be paid. Some cost sharing in such premium increases will be needed to avoid strategic behavior in which individuals claim to be high risk to get a higher credit. But a fairly modest sharing of the cost of additional premiums should suffice.

The fallback insurer receives no direct subsidy from the government and is permitted to risk rate its premiums. This means that there should be little danger that unusually costly risks within risk-rated categories will be shifted to the fallback plan, since the fallback plan will be charging them a price that will yield a competitive profit. If the fallback insurer can make a profit, so can other competitive insurers; "cherry picking" in our plan (in contrast to plans with full community rating) will actually reduce an insurer's profits.

The design of arrangements to deal with the risk of becoming a bad risk—and therefore facing higher premiums—is a problem in insurance specification. Risk-averse people would want to be insured against the future risk of unusually high premiums; variation in tax credits is a way of providing social insurance against that risk. Viewed as insurance, these policies should have the same features as other desirable insurances. They should not provide complete protection but should instead cover major threats to disposable income; they should be designed to avoid unnecessary administrative complexity; and they should distort other incentives as little as possible.

Risk-rated Credits and a High-Risk Insurance Pool. Whether limited guaranteed renewability will work without substantial administrative costs and distortions of its own is an open question. An alternative supplement to imperfect risk rating of credits is to establish a high-risk pool. Such pools permit individuals with designated high risk conditions who have been quoted premiums in excess of some multiple of a standard rate to obtain coverage at premiums that are somewhat higher than average but are less than what insurers would have charged. The pool can be subsidized either by explicit taxes and transfers (which would be our preferred solution) or by assessments on all insurers and self-insured groups offering standard coverage (which is equivalent to financing the subsidy with an excise tax on insurance purchases by standard risks).

The need for high-risk pools, however, would almost certainly be less under our plan than under the status quo for two reasons. First, as discussed, many of those with high cost conditions would qualify for greater income-related tax credits, both because poor health correlates with low income and because these income-related credits will be supplemented by some degree of risk-related credits based on objective indicators of expected high cost. These indicators will include age and a list of some objectively verifiable medical conditions.

Second, because coverage is mandatory, the risk of adverse selection will be lower, and insurers will have less incentive to incur underwriting expense to screen out higher-risk individuals. Insurers need to base premiums on risk to avoid adverse selection. With adverse selection impossible in RNHI, this need no longer exists. There is still an incentive to expend resources to identify *known* low risks to be able to attract their business by offering them lower insurance premiums, but there is no longer any need to identify high risks to prevent them from buying extensive coverage that they are almost sure to use.

Existing high-risk pools for health insurance are typically mandatory risk pools in which all commercial insurers writing health (and sometimes other lines) in a state must participate. The administration is handled by a lead carrier, but the deficits are allocated among insurers in proportion to their voluntary premium volume. In some states these deficits can be written off against premium taxes or other taxes.

An alternative is for the government to contract with a commercial insurer, on the basis of competitive bidding, to operate as an insurer of last resort. Although the same insurer might act as both high-risk insurer and fallback insurer, the relevant financing should be kept quite separate to prevent policyholders in the fallback insurer's basic business from subsidizing the high risks.

Assuming competitive contracting for a carrier for the high-risk pool, the difficult question is how to finance the inevitable deficit if rates are regulated below actuarial levels, without undermining the insurer's incentives to control costs. A simple stop-loss reinsurance arrangement in which the government bears all costs above the threshold is clearly nonoptimal. Some risk-sharing contract may be preferable. Financing the deficit through tax revenues is preferable to the more common current alternative of allocating the deficit prorata among all insurers, with or without a tax write-off.

Community Rating. An alternative approach for reducing the extent to which premium costs, net of government assistance, turn on risk factors is to require all insurers to practice some sort of community rating, that is, to require that individuals known to have different risk levels be charged the same premium. Several degrees of community rating are possible. At one extreme, full community rating would require uniform premiums for all individuals. This is objectionable on two grounds.

First, full community rating would increase insurers' incentives to select preferred risks (cream skimming), unless it were combined with strong regulation to ensure completely open enrollment and uniform rates for all insured people. With unrestricted competitive risk rating, insurers have no reason to reject high risks since they can charge an adequate rate, and they have no incentive to market aggressively to low risks because rates for low risks will be bid down to competitive levels. By contrast, under full community rating, insurers necessarily lose money on above-average risks and make a profit on below-average risks; thus, their incentive is to skim low risks and to avoid high risks. Vigorous regulation would be necessary to counteract the resulting selective marketing practices and would be unlikely to be fully effective.

Second, although community rating has a superficial appearance of equity, it is, in fact, a hidden and arbitrary tax—hidden because the young and healthy would be paying for the health care of the sick and older part of the population without explicit statement of this and arbitrary in that it would be paid without regard to ability to pay. Under community rating, subsidies to high-risk individuals are effectively financed by an implicit tax (premium above cost) paid by low-risk individuals, regardless of their respective income status and ability to pay, who happen to be covered by the same insurer. It is by no means true that all high-risk individuals are poor or that all low-risk individuals are well off. The inequity is exacerbated, in a way that cannot be offset by income-related tax credits, if the implicit tax on low risks and the subsidy to high risks depend on the relative number of sick and healthy individuals in each insurance plan. Community rating with multiple insurers does not tap all community members. The only way to have equitable community rating is to have only one insurer, but such a monopoly would have adverse consequences of its own.

Adjusting Premiums and Credits by Actuarial Categories. The disadvantages of full community rating could be reduced by permitting such rating only in the form of risk-related actuarial categories based on a set of objective predictors of expenditures (such as age, family size, and perhaps the presence of certain diseases). Health plans could be permitted to vary premiums by these broad predictors but not by other indicators of individual health status; individuals in a particular actuarial category in a particular area would be charged the same premiums for a particular plan.

This would reduce but not eliminate the cross-subsidization inherent in community rating; the narrower the bands, the less is the cross-subsidization. Since the plans would be prohibited from varying the premium within an actuarial category by health status, however, some cross-subsidization from the healthy (or the person who uses fewer health care services) to the sick or heavy user would remain.

Under any type of community rating, health plans must be required to accept all applicants who meet the categorical requirements, regardless of health status. The costs attributable to individuals with conditions requiring expensive treatment would be distributed across the members of the group in the actuarial categories into which they fell. Tax credits would be varied by the same actuarial categories used for premium rating. The actuarial categories could be adjusted to reflect those activities that increase utilization of health services and that society believes should not be cross-subsidized by others. Thus, depending on the political decisions, insurers could be permitted to modify the broad actuarial categories to reflect the increased costs of specified behavior, such as cigarette smoking or motorcycle ownership. Similarly, if society determined that this would be beneficial, insurers could be permitted to adjust the broad actuarial categories to reflect the different utilization patterns or risk characteristics of various professions. In this way, premiums would reflect a blend of broad risk factors (how broad would depend on the political decisions) without requiring an individual within a category who had actually become sick to pay a higher premium than others in that category.

This approach may be criticized on the ground that it reduces incentives for individuals or their employers to engage in health promotion activities. People do, however, have other incentives to keep well that are far more powerful than avoiding increases in the amount of their insurance premiums because of their health status; the question is how much difference a financial incentive makes to behavior. Employers' efforts to promote the health and well-being of their employees are also not likely to be affected if the group is self-insured or experience rated.

Conclusion. To the extent that the set of categories that insurers would want to use for risk rating differs from the set of categories that the

41

government wants to permit, the disadvantages of community rating remain to some degree. The real issue here is an empirical one: how divergent would insurers' preferred categories be from those the government would choose? In practice, the degree of fine-tuning of tax-credit categories involves a trade-off between the administrative costs of fine-tuning the credits and some residual unfairness if insurers use finer rating categories. It may well be optimal to permit some within-category variation in premium costs to individuals because the administrative costs of eliminating it are too great.

Remaining unanswered is the question of whether there really will be a serious problem, either of unfairness or of regulatory burden, under any of these approaches. The simplest policy would be to use the least interventionist option initially—that is, full and free risk rating for insurers—but to permit individuals to claim some adjustment of tax credits. Requiring limited guaranteed renewability of coverage at standard class rates for individuals and small groups could be a condition of the required coverage for all basic plans, so that the problem of high premiums or unavailability of coverage for high risks would diminish over time. But if experience should indicate that, even then, high risks still face unacceptably large differences in after-tax premium costs or that administration of risk-related tax credits is difficult, some regulation to create actuarial categories and to require more uniform rating within these categories could be introduced. Regulation should not be imposed until it has proved necessary. Heavy regulation to prevent a small amount of risk selection is unlikely to be cost-effective, may be hard to reverse, and may undermine potential efficiency gains from competitive insurance markets.

Most important, it would be inappropriate policy to hold coverage reform and the benefits of competitive markets hostage to the threat of what may amount to a modest amount of uncompensated risk rating or preferred risk selection, given the protections we have suggested. The benefits of competition outweigh the costs of troublesome risk selection; a monopoly national health insurance scheme would avoid the problem but at a heavy cost in efficiency.

7
Effects of RNHI

Adequate Coverage for All

RNHI guarantees adequate and affordable insurance coverage for all. Other strategies, such as the Pepper Commission proposal or the Enthoven-Kronick plan, which rely only on subsidies to induce nonemployees to buy coverage voluntarily, have two defects: they necessarily end up paying subsidies to people who would have bought coverage anyway, and they surely would leave some of the population uninsured. Our approach imposes an obligation to be covered and uses the tax system, supplemented by welfare agencies, to ensure that all receive appropriate coverage and subsidies so that all can pay their medical bills. It will also guarantee that workers will continue to be covered even if unemployed, with the premium net of subsidy during those periods geared to their income.

Requiring coverage implies restricting individuals' freedom to remain uninsured. Given the potential social ramifications of such decisions, however, the benefits of this restriction outweigh the costs. As a society, we already restrict individual choice and require insurance against costs of retirement and disability (social security), automobile accidents (mandatory automobile insurance in many states), workplace injuries (the workers' compensation system), and unemployment. These programs effectively mandate minimum coverage and leave individuals free to purchase supplemental coverage. The same logic should be applied to medical care and health insurance.

Minimal Disruption of Current Arrangements

Our approach does not disturb existing insurance arrangements for the great majority of Americans. Polls consistently show that Americans are dissatisfied with the health care system as a whole but satisfied with (though fearful about) their own situation. Most Americans have insurance at least equal to the minimum level of coverage that we envision. They usually receive this insurance through their employment. Although our proposal places the requirement to have insurance on the individual, it does not require each person to buy insurance individually; insurance may be purchased through an employment group, and employers will have strong incentives to select plans that best meet the preferences of their employees. The replacement of the open-ended tax exemption by a predetermined tax credit should be a powerful stimulus to employees and benefits managers to make efficient choices among insurance plans that meet the minimum standards and to make cost-conscious choices of supplemental benefits.

We anticipate that most medium- and large-size employers will offer several options, in the form of both fee-for-service and managed-care options, that provide the required minimum benefits. Within this framework, differences in copayment and stop-loss can easily be accommodated. Supplemental coverages might also be offered through employers. We also anticipate that group coverage will become increasingly available from other sources, such as banks, that can take advantage of administrative savings in premium collection; individuals who do not obtain coverage through employment will therefore face much better opportunities than they currently do.

Satisfying Individual Preferences

This plan permits arrangements tailored to differences in needs, tastes, and resources of individuals. No one structure for delivering care or method of reimbursement is best for everyone. Our scheme fosters diversity by locating the initial obligation to buy coverage with individuals; by permitting the individual to discharge that obligation through employment-based insurance, private purchase, or use of the fallback insurance; and by placing only minimum restrictions on services covered and out-of-pocket costs.

Greater Flexibility

Our approach provides maximum flexibility in the amount and distribution of the subsidy and the ability to pinpoint the subsidy. Subsidies to encourage coverage may be either more or less generous than the amount needed to achieve an equitable distribution of after-premium income. In our arrangement, the law mandating coverage can be tailored to achieve the desired level of coverage, by income class. Tax credits can then be used to offset the premium costs for this coverage in a way that yields a distribution of net cost that can meet the consensus notion of equity. From an economic viewpoint, we cannot define what is equitable; that is a design question for the political process. But whatever is decided can be easily implemented (and changed) within the framework that we suggest.

Removal of Existing Distortions

The current tax treatment of health insurance strongly subsidizes insurance in the employment setting. By eliminating the open-ended exclusion and replacing it with a fixed, income-related credit calculated independently of how much insurance coverage or medical care a person buys, we ensure that price signals reflect true resource costs. Individuals' insurance-purchasing decisions will not be distorted by the tax subsidy of the current system.

Distortions associated with mandated "employer-provided" insurance are also avoided. Requiring one to purchase some service for public benefit is formally equivalent to financing a public expenditure with a head tax. But in the case of health insurance, which is favored by the current tax exclusion, the financing is even more regressive than a head tax. The well-to-do actually pay less, net of taxes, than those with lower incomes. Moreover, much of the cost of mandated benefits ultimately falls on workers in the form of lower cash wages or fewer jobs. Mandated employer coverage will, in the first instance, cause employers to desire less labor, which will depress either money wage rates or employment. The analysis is complex and uncertain as to how costs will ultimately be distributed among employers, consumers, and employees, but the best bet is that the bulk of the cost will fall on employees. Since the added cost is proportionately greatest for the lowest income workers, the employer is most likely to find these workers uneconomic (if the cost falls on the employer), or they will suffer the largest relative diminution in cash wages to offset the cost (if it is borne by the employee). Roughly a third of the cost, in addition, will be borne by federal and state governments, through forgone income and payroll taxes, as taxable cash wages are converted into tax-excluded health insurance; the governments bear a greater cost if the worker is not hired, in lost taxes on income and in increased unemployment insurance, welfare, and Medicaid costs.

Contrary to this analysis, however, some who are engaged in the political process believe that mandating employer coverage will make "rich" employers pay for health insurance. That belief, together with the hidden nature of government costs, offers a strong temptation to politicians to expand benefit mandates. Our approach puts the costs in the first instance on individuals, which is where they will end up in any event, but distributes that cost in a fair way. Politicians could still determine the required level of coverage. But we suspect that the obvious cost of "giving" people more coverage under our plan—which requires individuals to pay more for insurance or the government to provide greater assistance if the required level of coverage is raised—will lead to more rational comparisons of costs and benefits than maintaining the current open-ended tax exclusion or mandating that employers obtain coverage. In such schemes, the cost to employees and taxpayers is hidden.

8

Appropriate Cost Containment

Our proposal, in contrast to some others, does not contain explicit mechanisms to control or to set limits on cost. Instead, we take the fundamental view that if responsible and informed buyers face prices and incentives that cause them to take actual costs into account—as our plan will—they can be relied upon to make choices that reflect an appropriate balancing of costs and benefits.

Consumer Choice

Consumers' choices will, by definition, lead to the right rate of growth of cost. New medical technology may be so useful and helpful to health or comfort, and the value consumers place on health relative to other needs may be so great, that consumers will in fact choose a rate of growth in medical spending in excess of the rate of growth in real GNP, and in excess of politically defined expenditure targets. If this happens, so be it. In this scenario, "controlling cost" would do more harm than good. Lower expenditures for health care, after all, have no intrinsic merit, since they mean only higher expenditures on other goods and services—and the real question is whether those higher levels of spending on other goods provide more benefit than the health care benefits forgone.

While we cannot guarantee some arbitrarily low rate of growth, however, our proposed system contains subtle but powerful incentives to rein in excessive cost growth and to yield rates of growth that (other things equal) are likely to be lower than the rates seen in recent years. Some additional reforms that are not really part of national health insurance, such as computerization of claims, effectiveness research, and malpractice reform, may be useful regardless of insurance arrangements.

Is there an appropriate rate of growth? Health care costs adjusted for

47

the size and demographics of the population have been growing faster than real GNP, year in and year out, as far back as we have reliable data. This growth primarily reflects three influences, whose precise contributions unfortunately are not known.

First, health care input prices—primarily wages of health workers and net incomes of health professionals—have grown more rapidly than general prices in many years; health providers have had to increase wages to attract trained personnel to meet the growing demand for care. Some of this growth in input prices surely translates into higher final prices for health care services and goods. Second, the type or technology of care has been changing. Changing technology, in both a big-ticket or miracle-machine sense and in a little-ticket or more caring-time sense, contributes the most important part of growth in real expenditures. Finally, perhaps there has been some increase in waste, some change that leads to using more inputs to do exactly the same thing. Some waste is expected because of the tax subsidy. It is difficult enough to document the changes in cost of constant-quality inputs, and so far it is impossible to separate changes in intensity that reflect higher quality or more beneficial intensity of care from those changes that reflect pure waste.

The primary source of inefficiency in the health care sector, in our view and in that of many other economists who have studied it, is not the growth of pure waste, of useless or harmful care. Instead, the primary source of inefficiency is the consumption of new types of care that are somewhat more beneficial than their predecessors but substantially more costly.

Our proposal does not require some centralized determination of what type of care is worth its costs, or worth doing at all. Instead, it envisions that those judgments will be made by firms organizing various types of health plans (although the firms' managers should surely benefit from current government-sponsored research efforts to determine what care is really effective). At a minimum, the plan that tries to control cost will have to submit someone—either patient or health care provider—to more inconvenience or hassle. In many, perhaps most, cases the inconvenience will be worth the cost savings, but we want to leave it up to individuals to decide how much effort, red tape, out-of-pocket payment risk, and bad feeling to undergo to save money. If individuals decide that the savings are worth the cost, fine; but if they decide, at least for a while, to shell out more money to preserve tranquillity and easy access to the latest and best care, that is fine too—as long as they are paying the cost of those benefits in the form of out-of-pocket payment or additional premium. Supplementary

48

premiums for supplementary insurance are to be permitted, although neither encouraged nor discouraged.

Our proposal removes one of the strongest subsidies to inefficiency present in the health care system today. Why do major corporations wring their hands over their rising health care costs and then profess an inability to do anything about it? Would we tolerate the same sort of schizophrenia if they told us they were paying too much for some other input but were too timid to get tough with suppliers? Probably not, but we need to recognize that there is a reason for employers to play the milquetoast when it comes to health care costs. An employer that imposes additional inconvenience on employees to cut their health insurance premium costs and passes on those cost savings in the form of higher money wages will be returning dollars that are subject to tax—at up to a 50 percent marginal rate if payroll and state income taxes are taken into account—but will be forcing the employees to lose 100 percent of the benefit of the medical care spending. No wonder that the employer and employees are still squeamish about aggressive cost containment.

Our proposal radically changes this calculus. Medical care spending under our proposal is subject to tax at the same rate as money income spent for other purposes; medical care spending and other spending will now all come out of after-tax income. Consequently, saving a dollar on medical care spending now will return exactly one dollar to the employee for spending on other things. The applicable economic theory is straightforward: by substantially increasing the reward from cost containment (nearly doubling it in locations with high tax rates), one would expect substantially greater efforts to be made. Not only would managed care be expected to flourish, but also corporate benefits managers might be expected to become more aggressive about making that managed care effective.

Research on managed care shows it thus far to be quite ineffective by itself in controlling the rate of *growth* in health care costs; managed care does produce a modest one-time cost reduction, but that decline soon gets swamped by a long-term trend of the same high real rate of growth as in the unmanaged care sector. What our plan promises to promote is not just managed care but *permanently effective* managed care—and it will do so precisely because high rates of real growth will always cost employees, who are responsible for the premiums, one hundred cents on the dollar every year.

This vision of effective private cost containment is still just that, a vision. But it is important to remember that a real competitive approach has never been tried, because the tax distortions did not make it worth the effort and because the traditional structure of the health care delivery system made it difficult to introduce. Providers competed not on price but instead on prestige. The payment system, and ultimately the tax subsidy to the payment system, enabled these institutions to pursue these objectives. Remove the subsidy, change the incentives, and institutions will either change their objectives or fail to survive.

Effects on the rate of increase in medical expenditures, by themselves, are not appropriate measures of whether market competition has worked or which country's health system is preferable. Allocating a given percentage of GNP for medical care is an inappropriate way to determine how much this country should spend on medical services. Allowing the government or health professionals to determine which services should be available to certain population groups (because they receive government assistance) or indeed to all Americans bases the value of those services on the judgment of those who are not affected or who gain financially from the choices. Considerations other than the value to the user, such as the political consequences of raising taxes, will affect expenditure decisions.

There is no better basis for judging the value of a service than the willingness of a person to pay for that service, provided that willingness is amplified for low-income people by means of tax credits. As long as medical services are produced efficiently and consumers are willing to spend their funds on medical services, then the resulting increase in medical expenditures is appropriate, regardless of how great it is.

"Can't Say No"

Henry Aaron has recently argued against the proposition that costs can be controlled to appropriate rates of growth by proper competitive markets.[11] He alleges that in a pluralistic society there is a fundamental inability or difficulty of denying anyone any service available in the market that patients demand and doctors are willing to recommend. He also argues that managed care would be powerless to restrain the use and growth of such services since neither the conventionally insured patient nor the fee-for-service physician faces any incentive to hold back from services of small benefit and high cost in the "main" market. For this reason, he advocates a publicly controlled single-payer system with private insurers relegated to administrative roles.

Part of his argument for this proposition is an inappropriate generalization from recent experience. Medical expenditures have increased consistently in the past few years, much as they have for decades before. It is unclear why Aaron thinks that this fact, in itself, proves that there is a problem. There were, after all, little or no additional incentives in recent years to control an increase in expenditure accompanied by an increase in quality since tax subsidies have not been reduced and in some ways have been made more stimulative with the new opportunity for tax-avoiding flexible spending accounts. The reduction in marginal federal income tax rates has been substantially offset by increases in federal payroll tax rates and in the maximum taxable wage subject to payroll taxes.

Moreover, the growth of real income per capita would in itself be expected to increase desired medical quality (and to fuel the demand for new technology); it is possible that medical care quality may be what economists call a luxury good, one whose demand naturally increases more than in proportion to income. (This term does not imply frivolity.) A growing share of income spent on such a good is consistent with proper market functioning. To be sure, no good can be a luxury good forever without eating up all income, but goods can be luxuries for quite a long time.

Aaron's major argument, however, is that in competitive markets the only possible constraints are demand-side constraints, which in health care are either too ineffective or too odious to be used as acceptable cost control devices. He argues that people will use whatever advanced technology is developed. Our view is that demand-side constraints do work. The full set of managed-care arrangements, moreover, is by no means limited to patient cost sharing. In particular, managed-care organizations can and do implement the supply-side strategy of reducing the marginal revenue that physicians would receive from providing or recommending additional services.

A competitive HMO cannot unilaterally decide to pay its doctors lower fees per unit of service, as the Canadian and German plans have done. It must compete for doctors, so their utility (involving both money income and working time) must be at least as great as they could get under fee for service. An HMO, however, can put physicians on capitation or put them at risk for some part of total costs (for their own or referred services); some of these devices do work.[12] A staff-model HMO that controls its own hospitals (such as the Kaiser plans) can be made aggressive. It can, if it chooses, limit both technology and budget. Malpractice issues aside, a Canadian provincial government can do nothing that the Kaiser health plan is unable to do. To be sure, in Canada the provincial monopoly is not

51

constrained by the competition as Kaiser is. Kaiser may be unwilling to cut costs and technology so deeply because it knows that the lower premium that such a strategy would allow is not enough to compensate potential enrollees for the loss of the latest technology. But that inhibition just demonstrates the point: competitive arrangements are better for determining what people really want than governments are.

As long as the market is large enough to allow the emergence of several such plans, unitary government control is unnecessary; competing plans can do every legitimate thing that government control can do. Plans cannot push compensation to nurses, doctors, and other health professionals below the competitive level, while a single government purchaser is able to do that. But such a transfer of income from providers to consumers does not necessarily lead to more appropriate total real costs.

In smaller markets, the key question is whether à la carte choice of quality and intensity is possible. In such smaller markets, the functioning of competition among insurance firms may be somewhat inhibited. It seems unlikely, however, that cost growth could get inordinately out of line even in this setting—since new entrants could reap substantial gains.

We have argued that the private sector is able to control cost growth but so far does not want to do so (because it has not had the proper incentives). Aaron argues that the private sector wants to control cost growth but is forever unable to do so. We fail to see a ground swell of consumer enthusiasm, even in the horde of public opinion surveys on this subject, for substantially reducing benefits and new technology to save money.

Aaron's argument may have some force if courts refuse to uphold contractual limits on covered services, forcing all plans to adhere to some norm more generous than is appropriate. If binding contracts become impossible, however, the problem should be addressed by appropriate legal reform, not by establishing a government monopoly of insurance.

Monopsony Power or Government Control

Private cost-containment efforts can control the use of real services and real inputs whose benefits fall short of their costs. But a competitive private market will not be able to force prices paid to health care workers—whether doctors, nurses, or technicians—below the competitive level. In contrast, many public systems in other countries do control costs exactly in this way.

Paying someone less to do the same thing does not really control cost in the literal economic sense of making more goods and services available to everyone. It only transfers incomes away from producers and toward consumers but does not increase real resources.

We *could* make hospital costs a lot less, and probably have to sacrifice only a little quality, if we as consumers formed a buyers' cartel and forced nurse wages down. We as analysts would not regard the use of such buyer market power—monopsony—as legitimate. Conversely, we as analysts (or consumers) would not regard provider prices pushed above the competitive level, whether by physician cartel or hospital workers' union, as legitimate either. The ultimate desideratum here is a market for medical services in which neither buyers nor sellers possess market power, so that prices—for both inputs and outputs—are at the competitive level. The solution is a strategy to prevent the exercise of either buyer or seller market power.

Our concern about the inappropriate use of market power extends to government. To the extent that government uses its large market power in a pluralistic system, its public relations power, and its ability to enact laws (denied to all other participants in the market) to force hospitals and doctors to accept prices below the break-even or competitive-market clearing price for services to its clients, and to the extent that providers shift costs, government is engaged in a shell game. It is not really reducing cost but just shifting it from taxes paid to support the government program to an implicit tax in the form of inflated private health insurance premiums.

9

Responses to Potential Criticisms

Of course there will be criticism of the Responsible National Health Insurance plan. A number of potential questions are addressed below.

Will credits be too administratively complex?

Our proposal will be challenged on the ground that it is too administratively complex to vary the required minimum benefits or maximum out-of-pocket costs with income. By tying the enforcement of the minimum coverage requirement directly to the federal income tax system and the welfare system, however, the additional administrative cost of our proposal should be small. The same system that determines other income-related transfers also determines whether a person has coverage appropriate for his income.

There is sure to be some additional cost for determining incomes for poorer people who do not now pay federal income tax or receive federal transfers. This is an unavoidable cost of the effort to tailor subsidies to needs. Enlarging the income range over which free insurance is offered can reduce this cost, because it should be easier to determine that income is below some cutoff than to determine the exact amount of income. But the cost of this simplification is the cost of excessive transfers and inequity across income levels.

Standardization of policies may offer some advantage. Some standardization is automatically produced by designating certain policies as the minimum acceptable policies for certain incomes. The label "$50,000-a-year policy" carries a great deal of automatic information. There may also be some role for aggressive, standardized designation. "Latest technology," "prudent technology adoption rates," or "only highly cost-effective care" would have to be modified as advertising slogans, but they would convey a lot of information about what one could expect from any plan.

Nonstandard policies could still be sold, as could individual insurance. Some people will always reject what the fallback insurer offers in their area and will chose not to work for firms that have already selected their policy. Such individuals should expect to pay more for the custom-designed coverage of their choice. But the higher administrative costs they entail would indicate the ability of the market to satisfy even atypical demand; the cost would not indicate inefficiency.

Will employment-related insurance disappear?

Our proposal will also be criticized on the ground that employers will stop providing coverage if the mandate is put on individuals; employment-based group insurance will be wiped out and replaced with more costly individual insurance. This outcome is implausible, although some changes may occur. The elimination of the tax exclusion applies to the worker, not to the employer, who can continue to deduct insurance premiums as part of total compensation cost. Because the employer's cost is left unchanged by the new program and the employee's productivity is not changed, the introduction of our proposal should not cause the employer to reduce or eliminate coverage.

Would employees want the employer to drop or cut coverage and return the savings to them in the form of higher money wages? If employees could obtain coverage in employment groups at significantly lower cost because of the scale economies of employment-group coverage, then they would choose to continue such coverage rather than to switch to individual or other group insurance. Some employees, however, may prefer to receive less insurance, subject to the required minimum, and higher cash wages when insurance is not tax preferred. This would reduce the amount of employer-provided insurance, a desirable effect because it would reflect employees' decisions on the level of coverage made on a tax-neutral basis and would cause total medical spending to fall.

In the current arrangement, tax advantages are much more generously available for employment-related group insurance in the form of a tax exclusion that provides larger benefits to higher-income taxpayers. The tax exclusion distorts choices in two ways. First, it causes persons to choose unnecessarily lavish insurance coverage with less aggressive cost-containment features. Second, it induces insurance purchasing through the employment-related group mechanism rather than through alternative, possibly more efficient mechanisms. Eliminating these distortions will probably affect employment-based coverage somewhat, although the extent of that effect is difficult to predict.

Employment-related insurance groups will probably remain the most efficient way for most Americans to purchase health insurance. As with any other economic arrangement, employment-related group insurance has its pros and cons. The problem with the current arrangement is that the tax subsidy overemphasizes the pros and leads to overuse of this device. Linking insurance availability to the job inhibits the efficient functioning of labor markets—the appropriate matching of workers to employment opportunities and job switching. The risk of losing access to tax-subsidized coverage if one quits and tries to take a new job affects workers' decisions about changing jobs. Moreover, buying insurance at the same place one sells his labor—the best arrangement for many persons—is not ideal for all. The people with whom one is grouped at work may not want the same type of insurance.

Our arrangement removes this distorted incentive to obtain insurance through the employer. It will probably result in some small firms' discontinuation of group coverage. It will have two important offsets, however. Many firms, especially large ones that can offer the most efficient form of group coverage, will definitely *not* drop coverage. Moreover, some small firms currently not offering group coverage will be induced to offer it, because their employees will all be obliged to obtain coverage and may well find the employment relationship to be the cheapest way to do so.

It is simply wrong to imagine that exclusion of the value of insurance from employees' wages is essential to the offering of group coverage. The recent experience with private insurance in Great Britain and New Zealand, mostly employment-group and all unsubsidized, proves that exclusion is unnecessary to induce employment-based group purchases. More important, it would simply be illogical for a large group or a large union to drop coverage and thus force workers to obtain the required insurance on an expensive individual basis. Large group insurance is likely to remain much cheaper than individual insurance.

A price must be paid for this mass marketing; individuals have to settle for the same insurance as some or all of their fellow employees choose. But particularly for the standardized basic coverage, such uniformity may not be onerous. If employment-group insurance remains so much cheaper, an employer who drops group coverage would be forcing the employees to pay more for a service the employer is already providing. That would not be a cost-minimizing compensation policy.

It is important to note that we are proposing only that employees be taxed on the value of group insurance paid for by the employer and that the obligation to secure coverage ultimately falls on the individual. We are not proposing that each individual employee be empowered to dictate whether or not coverage comes with the job or to choose whatever coverage he wishes. The employer or the union could, as at present, require that the employee accept reduced money wages to make a contribution to all or part of a health insurance premium as a condition of employment—and could refuse to contribute to insurance for someone who bought insurance elsewhere. Buying insurance could remain part of a job's essential conditions, like having a car to call on customers or investing in a business suit. But this requirement is not oppressive to workers, precisely because it would be adopted only when it offered a much lower price for health insurance. The employer or union, in other words, could choose the degree of compulsion about insurance purchasing that would be attached to a job—and would presumably choose that level most valued by workers in the labor market. In effect, by choosing to work for a firm that offers cheap but compulsory health insurance, workers would be constraining themselves for their own good.

More specifically, *RNHI neither requires nor encourages the purchase of insurance on an individual rather than a group basis.* It does place the obligation to obtain coverage on the individual, but it is to be expected that most individuals will choose to discharge the obligation in the least costly way, usually in some form of group insurance. Where employment-based groups are best they will be chosen, but we expect new sources of group coverage to emerge. Persons who fail to choose a specific group may also choose to buy coverage through the fallback insurer, which will take the form of a "group of last resort." That is, the fallback insurer should be large enough to offer most of the advantages of employment-related group insurance.

Even if rejecting the employment group were a possibility, the substantially higher administrative cost of individual insurance would make it unattractive even for good risks in large groups. In such groups good risks would not usually expect losses that differ substantially from the average—at least not by enough to make individual insurance attractive. It is currently possible to have tax-subsidized but risk-rated insurance, through the mechanism of flexible benefits or flexible spending accounts. Although there is no definitive information on the subject, we are not aware of any employment group that currently chooses to offer risk-rated insurance. This suggests that the administrative costs and the greater risk of jumps in premiums associated with such insurance do not generally offset the cost saving of conventional group insurance with premiums that vary only with family size and occasionally with employee age.

For smaller groups the price advantage of group over individual insurance is lower, as is the ability of groups to pool the high cost of above-average risks. If people differ in their demands for some aspects of insurance, group insurance may cease to be attractive to all members of the small group. In such cases either individual insurance or groups formed on bases other than employment might become a preferred option for some persons once the tax subsidy to employment-group insurance is removed. Some sets of employees will surely find that they prefer buying insurance in ways alternative to purchasing it as a tie-in sale with labor. In such cases, however, group insurance would no longer be the best option anyway: any cost advantage is offset by disadvantages, and the individuals will get the appropriate coverage in any case. In short, under our proposed reform, group insurance would disappear only when it was relatively less efficient anyway.

For firms that currently do not offer group insurance to their employees *and* that have relatively many uninsured employees, our plan would obligate the employees to find coverage. In many cases the least costly way of satisfying the obligation to obtain coverage would be to arrange it through the employment relationship. For the currently uninsured who do have an employed family member, the new obligation to buy coverage may create a new market for employment-group insurance. This new market may be sufficiently large that, on balance, the total size of the employment-group insurance market might grow.

There is therefore no reason to expect a substantial change in the size of the group insurance market, but there may be some dramatic and efficiency-improving readjustments in the identity of people buying insurance in this way, and in the form of the insurance they buy. Fundamentally, our plan establishes incentives to individuals to choose the best way to satisfy their insurance obligations, be it through employment-related group coverage, group coverage formed on some other basis, or individual coverage. The fallback insurer would set a baseline on the price someone must pay. People may prefer other types of insurance to the bare-bones variety offered by the fallback insurer, but at least the obligation could be satisfied in a low-cost fashion.

A converse criticism is that employers not currently offering coverage will not be induced by our plan to offer group coverage, even though employees would prefer it. For the employer to arrange coverage—if employees regard the group-coverage option as preferable—nonpoor employees would have to be willing to accept lower cash wages or to pay the premium directly by turning some part of their wages over to the insurer.

There is no reason why the employer should not be willing to help arrange such coverage; the employer would not bear the cost. Indeed, once an obligation to buy coverage is in place, employers who do not currently offer insurance might well choose to do so, if employment-based coverage is indeed more convenient. The only exception would be for workers at the minimum wage, if they were not permitted to exchange lower cash compensation for insurance benefits. Many of these individuals, however, would receive free coverage or would be covered by others in their families.

Wages should be defined to include insurance contributions. This prevents minimum-wage laws from barring low-income workers from employment-based insurance when it is most efficient. Such a change would simply recognize that the minimum wage should be defined in terms of total compensation.

Can individuals be trusted to choose their own health plans?

RNHI gives each person the obligation to obtain health insurance and the ability to pay for it. Advocates of conventional national health insurance may decry such empowerment of individuals on the ground that this usurps a proper role of the government, because individuals either cannot or should not choose their own insurance.

If there is to be a choice of which insurance to provide and what it will pay for, then someone must make that choice. The cornerstone of the American society and economy is that individuals make their own consumer choices. Individual choice is essential to reflect adequately people's differing desires concerning how their health care is delivered and what proportion of their resources they wish to allocate to it.

Individuals already choose their insurance in many instances and their providers in most. Giving more people the financial ability to make that choice does not change the basic arrangement for providing health care. It simply extends the right of choice now available to most of the middle class to the poor and other beneficiaries of government programs.

Individuals could choose to be aggregated into groups by employment, by membership in other groups, or by brokers and agents. This would enable them to exercise the collective purchasing power and expertise of the group—as they do now. For example, benefits managers could screen the options and even make the choices for those workers who wished to delegate this task. Our plan does not require individuals to make their own specific choices, but rather permits them to do so. Consultants who have expertise in picking good plans should find individuals and firms beating a path to their door.

The criticism that individuals should not be allowed to make their own choices implies that government should always make them for people and will make them better. There is no reason to believe, however, that real-world government can make these decision better than individuals. Government cannot reflect the individual desires of 250 million American people. Individuals who continue to obtain their insurance in connection with employment will be able to rely on benefits managers and benefits consultants to screen options and to help distinguish alternatives.

RNHI would provide more consumer protection than would the current system. A tax credit would be available only for the purchase of an insurance policy that met minimum standards and was geared to the individual's income. This would reduce the chances of fraud. In selecting a fallback insurer, moreover, the government would presumably act as a well-informed and prudent purchaser. State regulatory authority over providers would continue to protect quality.

Finally, since purchase of a qualified plan is required, at worst a poorly informed or inattentive buyer would pay more than he needed to pay for insurance. He would not go without coverage, and he would not purchase bad coverage. He would always have the option of the competitively bid fallback coverage as a reasonable insurance at a reasonable premium.

Can competitive insurance plans control the growth of medical costs?

RNHI does not seek to control the growth of medical costs as an end in itself. As discussed, cost growth has historically been caused by demographic changes, beneficial new technology, and the rise of medical input prices at a rate faster than that of prices in general. Our objective is to achieve a rate of future growth that represents an appropriate mixture of these factors.

We envision that competitive health care plans, offering various services to informed consumers, can achieve such a mixture. The main problem facing health plans will be that of choosing how much new technology to provide, and at what rate. At least some plans will have to ration beneficial but costly new technology. This hard message is dictated by an iron law of arithmetic: if real medical costs continue to grow at a rate faster than the rate of growth of real gross national product, then the fraction of GNP going to health care will grow without limit, and eventually all the real growth in GNP will go into medical care. Since such a biased allocation of resources is obviously not plausible, the rate of growth in medical costs will eventually have to slow. Since nothing can be done about demographic changes, the slowdown will have to come from one of two other sources: either from a change in technology or from a change in wages received by providers of medical inputs.

Any individual health plan is limited in its ability to affect the rate of growth in wages of health care workers. Individual plans, however, can in principle affect the rate of introduction and diffusion of beneficial but high-cost technology. One should not be overly pessimistic here; as the size of total expenditures grows, a given rate of growth translates into an increasingly larger absolute amount of beneficial new technology. Reducing the rate of growth could be accommodated by introducing a constant absolute amount of new technology each year. The problem is that, as yet, a reduction to even that level has not been achievable.

Two challenges face health plans in connection with new technology: one is related to choice, the other to heterogeneity. The challenge from choice is the requirement that the plan delay the adoption or slow the diffusion of new technology that provides definite medical benefits but at high cost. This is the only permanent way to slow the rate of growth in cost. Managed-care plans have historically said that they avoid only the care that is useless or harmful or that has lower-cost substitutes that are equally good.

The future challenge is to make choices when something of value must be sacrificed and to develop the discourse to communicate this idea to health professionals and potential plan members. *Someone* must make the rationing choice. The real issue is whether private-sector managers

61

have enough skill and nerve to do it themselves or will pass the buck to a public bureaucracy.

The challenge posed by heterogeneity will confront us if different plans are successful in controlling technology and rationally choose to do so. This will mean that some plans will be providing more beneficial care, at higher costs, than others. Such a situation will raise issues of acceptability and of legal standards. Unless we can find a way to tolerate such diversity of choice, however, there is little point in having a private market solution.

Physicians and hospitals will not be eager to enter the age of rationing for cost control. Some propose that effective competition cannot be obtained solely by the interaction of competitive plans: there must instead be one or a few super-buyer agents to consolidate market power to force providers to control costs.

Is such a quasi-regulatory arrangement necessary? Is market competition not enough? Market competition might not be best if providers have market or monopoly power, but this is unlikely to be the case in most metropolitan areas. Explicit or implicit collusion by hospitals and doctors to stonewall HMO or health plan efforts to introduce managed care are illegal under the antitrust laws, and they should be prosecuted as such. How many hospitals are needed for effective competition? Our judgment is that the real locus of competition is not the hospital but rather the physician and that there are enough physicians in all but isolated rural areas to permit effective competition. Some serious tasks will, however, have to be performed by hospitals. Either they will have to tolerate different protocols in the same institutions, or they will have to develop ways to separate the types of care they provide, so that they can simultaneously provide high-intensity and low-intensity care.

More vigorous competition will be found among health care providers in larger markets, just as it is with other goods and services. Except for the one-doctor town, however, in most places health plans should be able to offer choices. Even in the case of a single provider, a plan can always offer choices, and it can limit the provider's resistance by offering to transport insureds to larger market areas for nonemergency care or sponsoring a new entrant.

What if competition in competitive markets does not work to control medical costs? The simple but profound answer is that the costs should then not be controlled. If costs rise because the benefits from medical services justify the increase, then costs should not be controlled by regulatory measures.

Is RNHI politically unfeasible because it does not provide benefits to the middle class?

National health insurance is a visible political issue. The enactment of legislation that clearly redistributes wealth among the different income groups in society would typically require the support of the middle class. If the middle class is provided with large net benefits, however, then the total budgetary cost of RNHI would be increased and larger taxes would have to be imposed on some group other than the middle class to finance those benefits.

One means of financing RNHI would be to increase taxes on those with the highest incomes. Although this approach could be used for providing tax credits to those with low incomes, large tax increases would be required for those with high incomes if the middle class was also provided with generous tax credits. But there are an insufficient number of persons in the highest income groups to collect enough in increased taxes to provide tax credits to a large portion of the population.

One way to limit the tax increase for those with the highest incomes, while still providing benefits to the middle class, is to reduce the benefits going to those with the lowest incomes. The consequence of this policy would be either to limit provider participation, as has occurred in Medicaid, or to require those with low incomes to pay more out of pocket for their care. Either situation is undesirable.

Previously, legislative benefits for the middle class have been financed by regressive taxes on the working population. An example is social security financing for Medicare Part A—hospital services. A regressive tax to provide the middle class with tax credits is inequitable.

Thus, unless we are willing to accept a separate Medicaid-like system of delivery for the poor, to impose a regressive tax, or to require higher deductibles for those with low incomes, it would not be feasible to provide all members of the middle class—especially upper-middle-income families—with significant tax credits. Declaring employer payments for health insurance to be taxable income for employees would redistribute government subsidy on the basis of need to provide insurance for all. By definition the subsidy would be reallocated from families with higher incomes to those with lower.

Sizable numbers of middle-class families, however, would gain financially from replacement of the tax exclusion with a feasible tax credit.

Moreover, substantial benefits would accrue even to those families that pay positive net new taxes. There are also some misperceptions about what the middle class wants or can have that should be cleared away.

Let us deal with the misperceptions first. One relates to the preference mentioned above. Everyone would prefer a solution in which the health care system delivered the kind of care that insured, middle-class Americans receive today and did it for less per family than we spend now. Such an outcome is impossible. There is some inefficiency in the current health care system, but no method is yet available that would eliminate inefficiency and risk no harm.

Perhaps some method will eventually be found to curtail costly care that is harmful or of no value, and the incentives inherent in RNHI will encourage the development of such methods. Current federal and private research efforts to determine which care is effective and which is not will help as well. At the present time, however, no proven and generalizable method can do more for less. A great deal of experimentation occurs in methods of managed care, which often appear to offer only slight inconvenience or slight reduction in freedom of choice of provider or access to care in order to reap large cost saving.

But as yet there is no free lunch. Middle-class voters become woefully confused in the debate when politicians promise them something for nothing. Voters are sufficiently skeptical of such promises, however, to accept the facts as they are.

The other misperception is that the political process is assisted by designing systems of taxes and credits that can delude the middle class into believing that they will gain from some change. The most frequently suggested version of such a flimflam scheme is one in which credits are offered to persons at all income levels. The iron law of budgetary balance requires that any credits earmarked as medical insurance credits be offset by higher taxes of some type. If we confine ourselves to thinking about the federal income tax, then high credits for people at middle incomes and above would necessarily imply higher taxes for themselves or for upper-middle-income people. Neither political realities nor head counts indicate a sufficient number of very rich people to pay for an expense of this magnitude.

Politicians will try to highlight the credits and hide the additional taxes, but we place positive value on political transparency—on making it easy for voters to tell what they are getting and what they are paying for.

There is some room for adjustment here, as we will discuss in more detail below. Credits can be used to provide net benefits to the lower middle class, and the dividing line between those who receive positive net credits and those who pay for them will be determined by the political process. It remains an indisputable fact, however, that some in the middle class, especially those with incomes above the median, will have to pay rather than receive transfers.

Now we turn to what the middle class might expect to get from RNHI. It will be helpful to think of a concrete example: let us consider a system in which credits go to zero at a family income equal to 300 percent of the poverty line. In 1989 this would have represented an income for a family of four of approximately $40,000, which is in excess of the median family income. In the income class between 200 percent and 300 percent of the poverty line, as an example, the average value of the tax exclusion for families with heads under sixty-five has been estimated to be approximately $669, according to a study of the Department of Health and Human Services. The average unit in this income bracket would receive a tax credit, under a plan with a 300 percent-of-poverty maximum, of $697. Families in this income interval would experience a modest net gain on average.

This average, however, masks dramatic differences across families, depending on whether they formerly benefited from the tax exclusion or not. Families that formerly did not have access to generous, employer-paid health insurance or to any health insurance would gain if the exclusion were replaced by a credit. About 56 percent of families in this income interval would gain, with an average net credit among gainers of $518. In contrast, losers—those who formerly had generous employer premium payments—would suffer a net loss of taxes in excess of credits of $468. These differences among families at the same income level are stark testimony to the inequity of the current system of tax loopholes, in which nearly half the families at modest income levels get a substantial tax break that is denied to the other half.

At all income levels, with a plan that phases out the credit at 300 percent of the poverty line, HHS estimates suggest that about 41 percent of families, excluding families with only elderly members, would receive a net gain from an RNHI plan. Increasing the size of the cutoff modestly increases the proportion of gainers. It rises to almost exactly 50 percent at a cutoff of 400 percent of the poverty line and to about 57 percent at a 500 percent cutoff.

Some upper-middle-income families, however, would pay more in taxes than they receive in tax credits. What advantages would RNHI have for those families?

The first way in which upper-middle-class income families would gain is that RNHI would eliminate the cost shifting that results from the use of medical services by the uninsured. Some portion of the additional RNHI taxes simply represents more rational and more efficient ways of paying for care that low-income people would use anyway. The effect of eliminating cost shifting can be substantial, especially for those who buy insurance that pays charges. It has been estimated that the uncompensated care provided by hospitals, exclusive of any underpayment by Medicaid or Medicare, may amount to between 5 percent and 10 percent of total revenues. This burden varies considerably across hospitals, and it may be quite different for other medical services. Nevertheless, uncompensated care can be viewed as an excise tax on health insurance bought by the insured. If we assume that the average expense for potentially covered services is approximate $4,800 for a family of four and that cost shifting adds 10 percent, the implication is that the middle-class family's expected expense—premium plus out-of-pocket payments—could decline by as much as $480 after the passage of RNHI. This would offset a substantial amount of the increase in taxes.

There is a second immediate gain: the upper-middle-income family, and all citizens, would no longer have to be concerned about the underuse of medical services by the uninsured, especially the poor uninsured. The family would pay more in taxes per year, but it would get a clear conscience in return.

In responses to polls on the issue of the uninsured, Americans give apparently schizophrenic answers. On the one hand, almost without exception they lament the unfairness and undesirability of having some people without insurance being deterred from receiving beneficial care. On the other hand, when asked how much more in taxes they would pay to correct this inequity, they name figures that are unrealistically low relative to the likely cost.

These answers may simply be a manifestation of fiscal illusion; people want government to do many things they are unwilling to pay for. An alternative interpretation, however, would point to the absence of convincing evidence that there really would be substantial improvements in health if all were insured—because the uninsured currently receive some care. One can point to some selected medical services that the uninsured use less frequently than the insured that do have demonstrably positive impacts on health—such as prenatal care or hypertension screening. But there currently exists no basis for estimating how much good would be done by the spread of general insurance coverage. What would the tax-paying family be getting for its taxes in improved health indicators for its lower-income neighbors? At present, no one can say.

The main argument here is that the upper-middle-income family must become more persuaded than it is now of the need for and effectiveness of the additional care that universal insurance would induce. We think that this case can be made and that the middle class can be convinced that paying something for universal coverage is valuable.

There is a third and major reason why a middle-class family would benefit from RNHI: it would eliminate the currently distorted incentives that punish people who seek lower-cost health insurance plans. Our model family pays payroll taxes and income taxes, both federal and state. As a percentage of earnings, the marginal burden of such taxes can be as high as 25 percent. Higher-income families pay even higher marginal tax rates—up to 50 percent. Elimination of the tax exclusion would remove these distortions. But how would the family benefit from this?

Suppose the family is currently buying an old-fashioned, conventional insurance policy with low deductibles and nonmanaged-care, fee-for-service benefits. A managed-care plan may well be available to the individual family or to the firm, if something is sacrificed to join—a proviso that is common with such plans. The family may have to give up free choice of providers, may find the plan's contracted providers less convenient or more time consuming, or may worry about the chance of underprovision of care by a plan that makes more money the less it does. The plan may cost 30 percent less, however, than the old-fashioned plan.

Under current law, the family is punished financially if it selects the cheaper plan. Its taxable income would rise by $1,440—30 percent of $4,800—and its total taxes by $360—25 percent of $1,440—if it makes a choice that saves it and the economy a substantial cost. Small wonder if the family decides that the inconvenience is not worth the reward. In contrast, under RNHI the family would receive the full benefit of the cost saving, as its tax would be unaffected by the costliness of the qualified plan it chose. If it found a cheaper plan, it would pocket 100 percent, not 75 percent of the saving.

A fourth gain is brought about by the guaranteed coverage features of RNHI: indeed, guaranteeing coverage to all at affordable cost is the primary objective of RNHI. For a middle-class family, the most attractive feature of RNHI may well be relief from worry about losing coverage, for under RNHI that cannot happen. If the main earner in a family loses or changes jobs—in contrast to what sometimes happens now—coverage will continue. If income falls temporarily, then the size of the credit will automatically be adjusted, so the family will not be faced with a substantial premium increase to be paid out of an income shrunken to the level of unemployment benefits. If the family suffers a serious illness, then the combination of limited, guaranteed renewability and risk-related tax credits will keep coverage affordable. The requirement that the fallback insurer must accept all applicants will ensure availability.

There is another advantage of RNHI compared with a number of other national health insurance proposals. RNHI gives the family the freedom to choose the type of plan and the type of cost containment that it wishes, as long as it satisfies the minimum coverage requirement. In contrast, some proposals envision a single plan offered by the government or by a semiprivate corporation as the only choice, or the only subsidized choice, available to individuals. These plans are eerily like proposals to have health insurance provided by the post office, as a government-guaranteed monopoly—sharing the same danger of low-quality service, chronic deficits, and inflexibility.

The final potential gain from RNHI is more speculative, but it may be the most important. RNHI would encourage more cost-containing plans for individual or group buyers. The mere presence of an efficient, contracted fallback insurer would put pressure on costs. A large-scale movement toward managed care would do even more, as competitive pressures would affect even conventional insurance plans, and as the changed desires of health care plans and providers would change the kinds of technology that are offered.

If biomedical research firms know that innovations have to pass a cost-value test as well as a medical benefit test, they will do things differently. Moreover, as patient and plan demand pushes less strongly on the temporarily limited supply of medical resources, prices and incomes may fall. Nurses, for example, experienced a large rise in wages recently because of an increase in demand for their services. Lower demand would reduce the trend in which health care input prices, mostly labor but some supply and pharmaceutical costs, consistently run ahead of prices in general.

This roundabout way of pressuring doctors, nurses, technicians, and

68

producers of medical goods may appear to be less likely to succeed than heavy-handed government price controls or all-payer bargaining, but in fact it would be more appropriate. It would save more money if the benefits forgone were valued less than the cost savings, but it would not pursue cost containment for its own sake. RNHI would give the middle class the amount of cost containment it ought to have.

10
Comparisons with Other Plans

Three other approaches to health care reform can be compared with our plan: nationalized health systems, "Medicare for all," and play-or-pay (POP) plans. Some important differences exist between our version of market-based reforms and other proposals, such as that of the Heritage Foundation, which likewise proposes tax credits.

Nationalized Health Systems

The first alternative establishes a public monopoly of basic insurance. Representative Martin Russo has sponsored a bill of this form. Uniform coverage is provided to all citizens, with financing from general tax revenues, as in Canada and the United Kingdom. The claimed advantages of this approach are that it achieves universal and uniform coverage with administrative simplicity. But some advantages are more apparent than real, and there are real disadvantages.

The experience of Medicare and Medicaid, which are both public monopoly insurers for their targeted populations, indicates that administration is far from simple. Moreover, the experience under both these programs in the United States, as well as that under the nationalized health systems in Canada and the United Kingdom, is that individuals with varying preferences for medical care are dissatisfied with a monolithic, nationalized plan. A significant minority of British citizens buys private, supplemental, basic-services insurance—such purchases are prohibited in Canada—and a majority of Medicare recipients buy Medigap policies.

On the surface, these nationalized schemes appear better able to control the growth of health care expenditures than market or pluralistic strategies. The real social costs of these nationalized health plans, however, are severely understated, because the reported dollar expenditure figures do not reflect the time costs of patients and the forgone utility from unsatisfied demand that result from controlling costs by rationing the delivery of care. Nor do they reflect the tax-induced distortions of raising tax revenues to finance a nationalized plan.

Medicare for All

A modification of the Canadian approach has been proposed by Representative Pete Stark to extend Medicare to everyone. This scheme would provide a tax-financed, universal, and uniform basic coverage, with some out-of-pocket payments except for low-income families.

This scheme does permit private supplementation; the experience of Medicare has shown, however, that private supplementary insurance raises problems of its own. It increases the cost of the basic public program. It is often sold at very high administrative cost and in complicated forms, because it must be designed to fit around the complex public program. Although the low administrative costs of the public insurance alone are often highly praised, advocates fail to recognize that the high administrative costs of the supplementary insurance are an integral part of the cost of the whole system.

The fundamental point is that the level and type of insurance coverage people finally achieve under this system are unlikely to match the level and type they really want. It perpetuates the administered prices and government allocation decisions of Medicare. People may be able to cobble together a blend of private and public insurance that at least fits their preferences better than public insurance alone does, but the combination will never quite match their variation in taste for managed care, forms and types of coverage, and methods of administration.

"Play or Pay"

Perhaps the more realistic comparison for our plan is the other prototype approach. Its fundamental building block is a mandate that employers provide coverage to all employees and their dependents. Variants of this approach include the Minimum Health Benefits for All Workers Act, introduced in Congress several times by Senator Edward Kennedy and others; the Senator Jay Rockefeller-Claude Pepper Commission proposal, Access to Health Care and Long-Term Care for All Americans; the Massachusetts plan enacted in 1987 but so far not implemented; and the

71

bill written by Senator George Mitchell, HealthAmerica. Alain Enthoven and Richard Kronick have proposed a plan with a similar system of financing, but with a different emphasis on competitive health plans as a method of administration. We will first consider the legislative proposals and then turn to the Enthoven-Kronick approach.

Advocates of these legislative approaches claim that most uninsured people could be covered with no explicit additional government expenditure and without disturbing existing insurance arrangements for the majority of the population. None of these proposals, however, actually provides fully universal coverage, since a sizable minority of the currently uninsured are not in families with a full-time employed member. The advantages are overstated, and there are real disadvantages to this approach.

First, employer mandates typically exclude part-time workers; the Kennedy bill applies only to those who work at least seventeen-and-a-half hours per week and could cover at most two-thirds of the uninsured population.[13] If the mandate were limited further to full-time employees— those who work thirty-five or more hours per week—and their dependents, at most 54 percent of the uninsured would be covered. An exemption for establishments with fewer than ten employees would leave 60 percent of the uninsured uncovered. Cumbersome supplemental insurance mechanisms would become necessary, with supplemental sources of financing.

Second, these calculations assume that employers do not change their employment practice in response to the requirement. But in fact, there could be substantial changes in employment. If money wages do not fall sufficiently to offset the cost of insurance, employers either would substitute workers employed for fewer than the minimum covered hours or would employ fewer workers.

Third, the financing of an employer mandate is regressive; it is similar to a lump-sum or poll tax but with net tax rates that are actually inversely related to income, because of the tax subsidy. Among firms that finance their own insurance, the percentage that must be taken out of an employee's wage is the same where employees are middle income as where they are all well-off.

Fourth, the legislative employer-mandate proposals typically leave in place the current system of open-ended tax subsidy for employer contributions to health insurance. As we have argued, this system is inequitable and leads to excessive health insurance coverage, to use of medical care beyond the level justified by cost, and hence to excessive expenditure not only for medical care but also for insurance administration.[14]

Finally, although most persons are likely to choose the employment relationship as the basis for buying health insurance, there is no reason to favor this arrangement or to require it for all.

Some proposals add a supplementary scheme, sometimes with higher subsidies, to cover those who would not be covered by an employer mandate. This large subsidy is presumably motivated by the desire to achieve near-universal coverage without mandating it. The subsidy scheme introduces a horizontal inequity between the employed and those not employed, at the same income.

Some proposals, such as the Rockefeller-Pepper Commission's, would establish subsidies for certain small businesses to encourage them to provide coverage, while limiting the mandate to firms of more than 100 employees. Using a subsidy to induce coverage is inefficient, because the subsidy rate required to attract some will be more than enough to attract others, resulting in a waste of tax dollars. Moreover, in the case of a subsidy targeted at small businesses, there is the added objection that tax subsidies should be targeted at those in need. It is by no means true that all employers or employees in small firms have low incomes.

By contrast, our plan places the ultimate obligation for coverage on the individual rather than on the employer, with a uniform system of tax subsidies that depends only on the individual family's income and risk level, not on employment status. It thereby achieves universal coverage, eliminates horizontal inequities and incentive distortions between the employed and the unemployed, establishes a system of financing that is progressive rather than regressive, and closes the current inflationary, inequitable tax loophole. It offers neutral incentives to individuals concerning the choice between employment, group, and individual insurance. It protects the low-income worker from the unaffordable expense of having to pay for employer-provided coverage through a wage offset. It relies on the established insurance industry to provide a competitive product, and it provides for contracts between private insurance and the government as necessary to provide fallback insurance.

In practice, how would POP plans work? If the average wage in a firm is low, it would be better for employees and employer to have the employer "pay" the tax, because the total tax is less than the premium that would be required to "play." The cutoff between pay or play is that average wage income which, when multiplied by the tax rate, equals the actual premium cost for the required plan.

For instance, if the average premium cost for the required plan is

73

$3,000 per employee, averaging employee-only and dependent premiums, and the tax rate is 8 percent, then the cutoff income is $37,500. At this income level, an 8 percent tax collects $3,000, an amount just equal to the premium that would have to be paid. There is some ambiguity in the treatment of the employee contribution, especially at low income levels, depending on whether the employee is required to make such a contribution even if the group chooses the tax approach. We will ignore this in our discussion and assume that the alternatives for employees are to pay the premium in full, either by explicit payment or by reduction in money wages, or to pay the tax.

For employees in those firms that are constrained by the POP rules, the effect is much the same as if the minimum insurance coverage were obligated, employees were required to pay for it, and a tax credit or subsidy were provided at all wage incomes below the cutoff income, equal in amount to the difference between the premium and the tax. Since employees who choose to pay will pay less than the cost of their insurance, and since those who choose to play will just cover the cost of their insurance, we know that the plan will need a subsidy from general revenues. This subsidy will be distributed to those whose tax bill is lower than the true premium cost of the insurance they received. Viewed from this perspective, POP schemes are just a regressive special case of an RNHI-type tax credit arrangement.

There are some important limitations on POP schemes, however, that are avoided under RNHI:

• The tax-and-transfer mechanism under POP plans may not match what society would prefer. In net cost, the method of financing the required coverage in a POP plan is virtually identical to the way social security and Medicare have traditionally been financed, with a proportional payroll tax that reaches a limit at some cutoff income. Such a scheme is regressive, in that taxes as a percentage of income or wages decline as incomes rise above the cutoff level. In contrast to RNHI, POP schemes would impose positive premium payments even on very low-wage workers.

• The transfer under POP schemes is based on an employee's wages, not on his income. Thus persons from high-income families working low-wage jobs—that is, young workers, or workers who work just enough hours to be classified as full time—will receive transfers even though their family incomes may be quite high. By contrast, RNHI bases credits on family income.

• Most POP schemes envision a fairly generous insurance plan, with some additional generosity (or waiver of out-of-pocket payment) for very low-wage persons. Such coverage may well be excessively generous for some upper-middle-income families; RNHI, by contrast, tailors the amount of required coverage to the family's needs, rather than choosing one-size-fits-all.

• POP plans do not provide universal coverage; RNHI does. While the cracks would be narrowed under POP plans, some gaping holes would remain in the obligation to obtain coverage: part-time workers, persons who work for small firms, the self-employed, and persons in families who obtain no income from wages. Any employment-based system suffers from this important defect.

• POP plans perpetuate the fiction that the employer, not the employee, is paying for employment-related coverage. This arrangement offers the possibility of distorted political choice. By contrast, RNHI is specific and explicit about who will pay what—and about who will pay how much more if benefits are increased.

• POP plans rigidly link private coverage to the employment-related group. While that may be the ideal group for many persons, it may not be the best for all. Linking coverage to employment may mean that labor markets are distorted and that some persons end up in groups smaller, and with higher administrative costs, than those they would be in if they could choose to belong to larger groups associated with churches, schools, or communities.

• POP plans retain the exclusion of employer payments from taxable income, which fuels the inflationary fire.

• POP plans rely on government coverage for employees whose employers find it more economic to "pay" than to "play." This will create a massive government program, deprive the employees who are subject to it of choice and access to the private insurance market, and subject them to the coverage and allocation decisions of government. It is, indeed, not beyond the realm of possibility that the government could collect more in employer payments than it decides to devote to the health care of the individuals on whose behalf the payments are made.

The Enthoven-Kronick Proposal

The proposal by Alain Enthoven and Richard Kronick uses a play-or-pay financing mechanism and suffers from the defects of that mechanism. It offers a crucial structural improvement, however, over the legislative proposals: it limits the open-ended tax exclusion. Specifically, employers

75

would be required to make a fixed-dollar contribution for all employees. Any additional premium in excess of that contribution would be the responsibility of the employee. Employees would have to pay tax on any employer contribution in excess of 80 percent of the average cost of a qualified health plan in the employer's geographical area. Current methods of tax shielding in the form of flexible benefit plans or flexible spending accounts would be abolished.

This change accomplishes the same goal as the replacement of the exclusion by a closed-end credit under RNHI: it means that additional dollars spent on health insurance are not tax subsidized, so that employee choices will be efficient, cost-conscious choices. Both the Enthoven-Kronick plan and RNHI therefore pursue the same objective of improved incentives; the primary difference is that RNHI imposes fewer restrictions on the circumstances in which individuals make these choices, as RNHI does not require coverage to be provided in the employment setting or set rules as to employer contributions.

Other Tax Credit Approaches

Our scheme also involves less government intrusion and distortion than in the strategy suggested by the Heritage Foundation.[15] That proposal, like ours, places some insurance obligation on individuals. Unlike our proposal, it uses open-ended tax credits for both insurance premiums and out-of-pocket payments. The open-ended credit, which matches the consumer's expenditure at some percentage rate regardless of the size of the expenditure, is as inappropriate as the current tax subsidy.

Moreover, the plan envisions a higher percentage matching rate to favor out-of-pocket medical expenses over insurance coverage. The intent is to "encourage consumers to purchase routine services out-of-pocket," and presumably it would impose the administrative burden of reporting and monitoring of those expenses. In contrast, our approach provides a fixed-dollar tax credit, leaving consumers to make choices between insurance coverage and out-of-pocket payments, beyond the maximum permitted level, based on a neutral consideration of the true cost of each option and the benefit to each individual of risk avoidance. Our proposal is neutral between plans that use a supply-side strategy to control cost and those that rely on a traditional copayment approach.

Heritage's proposal also encourages "workers to purchase medical care and health insurance on their own" rather than through employment-related group insurance. The discussion of how this bias against group coverage would be accomplished is not detailed, but it is suggested that there be "legislation requiring employers to distribute among their employees the money they now spend on health insurance." Our proposal does not intrude on the employer-employee wage determination process, and it permits the use of employment-related group insurance by firms that expect that strategy to be attractive in the labor market.

Incremental Tax Credits and the Chafee Bill

Republicans in the Senate have recently proposed a set of new tax credits and a broadening of tax deductibility. Specifically, their bill proposes up to $1,200 worth of tax credits for expenditures by individuals with family incomes below $32,000 for health insurance premiums or out-of-pocket medical expenses, along with a temporary credit equal to 25 percent of premiums for small firms that cover employees or dependents through managed care. It extends income tax deductibility of premiums to those who do not receive employer-provided insurance.

Implementation of a fixed tax credit is a step in the right direction. The Chafee bill, however, falls far short of an integrated and substantive reform. It does not address the inflationary tax exclusion; indeed, it compounds the problem by extending the tax favored treatment of premiums to the rest of the population. And it does not require that individuals obtain coverage; it still tries to use subsidies to influence the behavior of those already shown to be resistant to subsidies.

The credits and extended deductions for premium costs it proposes, however, could serve as transitional steps toward an RNHI-type arrangement. Even extensions of the tax subsidy for purchase of health insurance can become the equivalent of tax credits, as we discuss below.

11
The Cost of RNHI

The implementation of an RNHI scheme would involve public outlays for the new tax credits. These outlays would be offset by lower public expenditures for the acute care provided by Medicaid programs and by other public programs for medical care for low-income persons or for former public employees, especially veterans. In addition, eliminating the tax exclusion by requiring employment-based insurance payments to be treated as part of income would increase collections without a change in tax rates. How these changes net out depends on the particular form chosen for providing RNHI-based credits.

Budgetary Studies of RNHI

Several studies have developed estimates of the net budgetary effect of some sample RNHI schemes. (These "costs" represent the public fiscal consequences of implementation of the plan; they are to be distinguished from the true cost of resources consumed.) All of these schemes take the form of defining a maximum tax credit for persons below some income level and then reducing the size of that credit in a linear fashion down to some income limit defined as a multiple of that income level.

Suppose, for instance, that the cost of the full coverage plan for a low-income family of a given size and age composition is $3,000, and suppose the poverty line for that family is $12,000 per year. Then a sample "300 percent of the poverty line" plan would offer credits of $3,000 to all families of that type with incomes below $12,000 and would reduce the size of the credit as incomes rise above $12,000, reaching a zero credit at an income of $36,000—or 300 percent of the poverty line. In this example the credit would be reduced by $125 for every additional $1,000 in income in excess of $12,000. Adjustments for family size, for high risk, for age, and for location would need to be made to develop an aggregate figure.

Our intent is to provide estimates that tie the definition of low income to the federal poverty line. A complication in developing such estimates is that the poverty line is linked to income in a family or household (as defined by the Census Bureau), while insurance premiums are linked to an "insurance unit" as defined by insurers, and taxes are linked to units as defined by the tax laws. Usually all three units coincide, but some households contain persons in different generations related in various ways for which there are differences. To take an especially complex example, a household with a head older than sixty-five, containing a daughter and grandchildren, may display "census household" income above the poverty line—but the daughter may report a low income for tax purposes.

Several estimates have been developed of the budgetary cost of RNHI schemes, differing in the ways that households are defined for purposes of determining eligibility for the low-income credit. Here we discuss results from a study done for the Department of Health and Human Services that uses the most fiscally conservative definition of a unit. It would treat the daughter and granddaughter in the example as a separate low-income household, entitled to a large credit or voucher. More precisely defined rules of eligibility could be expected to yield budgetary costs less than these estimates.

Budgetary Cost of RNHI

If all persons younger than sixty-five are included, the HHS study estimates the net federal budgetary cost for a "300 percent of the poverty line" plan, after considering the elimination of the tax exclusion but before incorporating tax deductions, Medicaid, and other expenditure cuts, to be $16 billion in 1991. This represents a gross cost of the credits of $71 billion, with the removal of the tax exclusion yielding $55 billion in offsetting federal taxes. Medicaid acute care costs for the population younger than sixty-five amounted to an estimated $30 billion in 1991, while other federal governmental medical costs were about $6 billion in that year. These figures suggest a net cost of a "300 percent" program of *negative* $25 billion. (The cost savings could be increased if the deduction in the individual income tax for medical expenses were also eliminated; that would save approximately $4 billion.) That is, an RNHI program of this size would save the federal and state treasuries a fairly sizable amount.

If we increase the cutoff income to 400 percent of the poverty line, this change both adds additional recipients of credits and increases the size of the credit paid to those already receiving credits. The net tax cost of such a plan is about negative $9 billion; the gross cost of the credits rises by $16 billion, to $87 billion. A 500 percent plan costs a positive $7 billion net. Within fairly broad limits, a plan with a maximum cutoff income in the range between 400 and 500 percent of the poverty line apparently would just use up all the additional taxes and expenditures savings; it represents the budget-neutral substitution of credits for elimination of tax exclusion. Such a 400–500 percent plan would provide a positive income transfer to a majority of individuals. Its primary cost would be somewhat higher taxes (in the neighborhood of about $800 per family) on upper-income and upper-middle-income families.

These estimates might be optimistic. They assume a minimal loading cost for insurance and do not include high-risk credits. Conversely, they do not envision the reduction in total medical spending expected from RNHI. As noted, such savings could mean that RNHI would increase income to be spent on other things for all but the most well-off.

While the RNHI plan does envision tax increases for upper-income families, those increases are smaller, by a substantial amount, than the gross taxes needed to finance plans such as the Heritage proposal that continues substantial tax credits for the well-to-do. A "500 percent" RNHI provides more generous credits for persons between 200 and 300 percent of the poverty line than does the Heritage plan, but lower or no tax credits for those who are further above the poverty line. A cutoff at 500 percent of the poverty line extends the tax credits up to an income level of $66,000 and provides positive *net* credits (credit less additional taxes on employment-provided fringe benefit) up to about 400 percent of the poverty line.

Even the modest "cost" of a reasonable RNHI plan represents only budgetary costs, not true economic costs in the sense of consumption of valuable resources. Most of the cost is in the form of transfers from well-to-do beneficiaries of the tax exclusion to lower-income families, the majority of whom currently buy coverage with only minimal tax subsidies. The uninsured already consume on average about 60 percent as much medical care as the insured. The *real cost* of RNHI depends on the extent to which the use of care will increase among the uninsured when they receive coverage. The real social cost of universal coverage that represents the cost of this additional care, plus additional administrative expense, is approximately $17 billion.[16] This amount is included in the tax costs discussed above.

12
Alternatives and Implementation

Alternatives to Eliminating the Tax Subsidy

Despite the efficiency and equity improvements that would follow from eliminating the tax subsidy for employment-based insurance, legitimate objections to removal of this tax advantage are raised by those who planned their employment choices and benefits policies on the existence of some type of exclusion. Are there ways of removing the distorted incentives and inequity among purchasers at each income level that would *not* require elimination of the subsidy?

One way to achieve this objective does have a cost in terms of higher tax rates. (It need not, however, increase the aggregate net tax burden.) The following scheme is suggested. Taxpayers would be permitted to exclude from their taxable incomes an amount equal to the estimated premium cost of the minimum coverage plan for their income level instead of electing a tax credit. They would be eligible for this exclusion regardless of how they obtained the insurance, whether through employer contribution or their own payment of premiums. The expected premium would be determined by what the fallback insurer in the area had bid for offering the required coverage. Tax rates would be increased, in some politically acceptable fashion, to accommodate any revenue shortfalls that this plan would cause.

How would this scheme work, and how would it differ from a system of tax credits only? For low-income persons, credits would almost always be selected because those persons get little benefit from a tax exclusion. Middle-income persons currently benefiting from the tax exclusion could choose to retain some of that benefit, and the benefit would be extended to persons at the same income level buying the same insurance who did not take a job with employer contributions. For incomes above the cutoff for credits, the exclusion would be preferred, and even some of those eligible

81

for small credits might prefer the tax exclusion.

Such a scheme would have a higher cost than a system of credits alone since it would never pay out less than the credit and sometimes would pay out more. The additional cost would depend on the generosity of the credit system (the size of the cutoff income) and the pattern of actuarial values of mandated coverage.

This scheme does achieve horizontal equity (by extending the tax subsidy to all). It achieves efficiency by capping the tax exclusion so that the value of the exclusion does not vary with the cost of the policy that a family actually selects; a family that chooses a lower-cost policy (down to the minimum) will be able to retain all its gains. In effect, this policy simply adjusts a person's federal tax, giving a reduction in taxes equal to the taxes that would have been paid on the excluded amount of income, but then adds whatever taxes would be necessary to fill the revenue shortfall.

Phased Introduction

Congress will need to consider whether to phase in RNHI. A phase-in might add complexity to the system and confusion for people and could jeopardize acceptance of the plan. A phase-in would reduce the "shock effect" that the introduction of a more competitive system should have on the health care delivery system. Introducing the plan in stages would reduce the extent to which it would stimulate the actions necessary to make the system more efficient and would lead critics to declare competition a failure before it had a chance to operate (as under the present system).

Nevertheless, if Congress decided to phase in RNHI, it could so gradually in various ways. Some provisions could be enacted immediately. The obligation to purchase insurance could be imposed first on individuals with incomes high enough that they would not be eligible for a credit. Most of these would already have qualifying insurance, and the cost of obtaining insurance for those who do not have it would be slight. The concept of required insurance would thus be introduced and imposed first on those who could satisfy it without government assistance.

Other components of RNHI could also be introduced without cost. State-mandated health benefits, such as those that require coverage of certain services (for example, hair transplants) and certain providers (for example, chiropractors), could be preempted immediately for all health insurance. Similarly, insurers could be required immediately to renew policies at standard rates or within a stated percentage of standard rates for a given time.

For political reasons, it might be difficult to remove the exclusion immediately from taxable income of employer-paid health insurance. Eliminating it completely and at once could result in a great deal of opposition from unions, health care providers, insurers, and others, although as we discuss above, the benefits to the middle class of the entire package could override concern over redistribution of the tax subsidy. If the compromise were to phase out the exclusion, the tax credit could be phased in as the tax exclusion was phased out. To do that, the tax exclusion could be capped. This limit could be set equal to what the required coverage costs from the fallback insurers or to what people with average incomes receive. This limit would not, however, be indexed against inflation. The tax credit would then be phased in on the basis of the "savings" generated by the cap on the exclusion.

13
Conclusion

The approach to national health insurance that we have outlined has emphasized responsible choice at several levels. It emphasizes the responsibility of all Americans to obtain insurance and of nonpoor citizens to pay for medical care services to the extent of their ability. It emphasizes as well the responsibility of consumers to choose whether they want to buy more comprehensive health care and health insurance or whether they want to spend their money on other goods. It emphasizes the responsibility of government in providing resources for low-income people to help them pay for the care and coverage they need, especially when their health risk is unusually high. It emphasizes the responsibility of the tax system to offer undistorted choices among insurance options and to close tax loopholes that subsidize generous health insurance for the well-to-do. And it gives the government an alternative to the tempting but misguided approach of employer-mandated benefits.

Exercise of these responsibilities provides a substantial benefit. It gives all citizens the opportunity for maximum informed choice. Our plan does not offer any magic way of cutting costs, any sure-fire scheme to deliver more for less, any easy way for employer benefits managers to pass the buck for rationing medical care, or any dream tax to allow politicians to finance medical services in an off-budget way. It does allow the greatest scope for consumers, within a competitive health care market, to compare the true costs and benefits of medical care, health insurance, and medical care plans and then to make the choices that will benefit them most.

Notes

1. Mark Pauly, Patricia Danzon, Paul Feldstein, and John Hoff, "A Plan for 'Responsible National Health Insurance,'" *Health Affairs*, vol. 10, no. 1 (Spring 1991), pp. 5–25.

2. The notion that ideal national health insurance should take the form of income-related catastrophic coverage has been advocated by health economists for twenty years. See Martin Feldstein, "A New Approach to National Health Insurance," *Public Interest* (Spring 1971): 93–105, and Mark Pauly, *An Analysis of National Health Insurance Proposals* (Washington, D.C.: American Enterprise Institute, 1971).

3. Delineations of the core services and of the maximum stop-loss are related. If the minimum set of core services is less than what most people would prefer, many will choose to incur additional expense, either out-of-pocket or in supplementary insurance. The less comprehensive the definition of core services, the lower the maximum stop-loss should be.

4. Another view of the system of subsidies for low-income and high-risk individuals to buy coverage is that it is a mechanism of social insurance against becoming high risk.

5. Randall Bovberg, Philip Held, and Mark Pauly, "Privatization and Bidding in the Health Care Sector," *Journal of Policy Analysis and Management*, vol. 6, no. 4 (Summer 1987), pp. 648–66.

6. Varying the credit by area would represent a departure from the usual tax policy since almost no provisions in the tax law vary with local conditions. The size of the exemption for dependents, for instance, is the same everywhere in the country, although surely the cost of raising a child across areas varies as much as the cost of medical insurance premiums. The closest one can come to geographic variation in tax policy is to note that when deductions were available for state sales taxes, tables with the different tax rates were used as the basis for deductions in lieu of proof of actual sales tax expenses.

7. If tax credits are adjusted for risk status, as discussed below, it may be necessary to gather information on the premium charged to this small proportion of the population. For all individuals, enforcement will require verifying that the insurance policies meet the conditions for a credit. This is like any tax credit and is really only an aspect of the rule that qualified insurance be bought. It requires a calculation of every person's credit as part of any necessary compliance review of selected individuals.

8. The model for doing so currently exists for employer payments for group life insurance in excess of certain values. Those excess premiums are reported in the worker's W-2 form and are to be added into taxable income.

9. Alain Enthoven and Richard Kronick, "A Consumer-Choice Health Plan for the 1990s," *New England Journal of Medicine,* vol. 320, no. 1 and no. 2 (1989), pp. 29–37, 94–101.

10. This is in contrast to the Heritage Foundation tax credit proposals.

11. Henry Aaron, *Serious and Unstable Condition: Financing America's Health Care* (Washington, D.C.: Brookings Institution, 1991).

12. Alan Hillman, Mark Pauly, and Joseph Kerstein, "How Do Financial Incentives Affect Physicians' Decisions, Resource Use, and Financial Performance in Health Maintenance Organizations?" *New England Journal of Medicine,* vol. 321, July 13, 1988, pp. 86–92.

13. Alan C. Monheit and Pamela F. Short, "Mandating Health Coverage for Working Americans," *Health Affairs* (Winter 1989), pp. 22–38.

14. Patricia M. Danzon, "The Hidden Costs of Budget-Constrained Health Insurance Systems" (Paper presented at an AEI conference, American Health Policy: Critical Issues for Reform, October 3–4, 1991).

15. Stuart Butler and Edmund Haislmaier, eds., *A National Health System for America* (Washington, D.C.: Heritage Foundation, 1989).

16. For more precise estimates, see Patricia M. Danzon and Frank Sloan, "Covering the Uninsured: How Much Would It Cost?" Leonard Davis Institute Working Paper 9, December 1986.

86

About the Authors

MARK V. PAULY holds the Bendheim Professorship and is professor of health care systems, insurance, public management, and economics at the Wharton School, University of Pennsylvania. He is director of research for the Leonard Davis Institute of Health Economics, University of Pennsylvania. Mr. Pauly received his Ph.D. in economics from the University of Virginia.

PATRICIA DANZON is the Celia Moh Professor of Health Care Systems, Insurance, and Risk Management at the Wharton School, University of Pennsylvania. She is an elected member of the Institute of Medicine. Ms. Danzon earned her Ph.D. in economics from the University of Chicago.

PAUL J. FELDSTEIN is professor and FHP Foundation Distinguished Chair in Health Care Management at the Graduate School of Management, University of California, Irvine. He earned his Ph.D. from the University of Chicago.

JOHN HOFF is a practicing attorney and member of the law firm of Swidler & Berlin in Washington, D.C. He is a specialist in health law matters. He received his LL.B. degree from Harvard University.